Legal Disclaimer

The author and Healthy Kidney Publishing are legally obligated to include this disclaimer due to the litigious nature of today's world, which may give rise to accusations, criticisms and attempts to suppress and discredit the work.

This book or guide and all the information contained in it are copyrighted with all rights reserved. The author, the publisher and anyone associated or affiliated with Healthy Kidney Publishing does not assume any liability for the misuse or use of information contained herein.

The content in this guide or book is provided for educational and informational purposes only. It is not intended, nor should be a substitute for, professional medical advice from a medical doctor, diagnoses or treatment. The author is not a medical doctor nor a licensed health care professional, nor does he claim to be.

Never disregard professional medical advice from a licensed health care professional or delay in seeking it, because of something you have read. Always consult your medical doctor or your primary health care provider about the application of any opinions or recommendations with respect to your own or someone else's symptoms or medical conditions.

Robert Galarowicz and Healthy Kidney Publishing and any of their websites, the author and anyone associated with them, shall have neither liability nor responsibility to any person or entity with respect to any loss, damage, or injury caused or alleged to be caused directly or indirectly by the information contained in this book, eBook or guide.

Every attempt has been made to provide information that is both accurate and proven effective; the author, Healthy Kidney Publishing and by extension the guide or book, make no guarantees that the remedies, nutrition, diet, supplements, testing, lifestyle changes and any information presented herein will help everyone in every situation. As the symptoms, diseases, conditions for each person are unique to the individual histories, body type, physical conditioning, medical conditions, and the specifics of the actual kidney disease, success will vary.

You should never stop taking any medication without first consulting with your medical doctor or health care provider. You should consult with your medical doctor or health care provider before beginning any health maintenance or improvement program.

All information contained and any links are for informational purposes only and are not warranted for content, accuracy or any other implied or explicit purposes.

This guide or book is sold subject to the condition that it shall not by way of trade or otherwise, be rent, lent, sold, hired out, given away or otherwise distributed without the author or publisher's consent.

Not one single part of this book, guide, and publication may be reproduced, edited, stored in a system or transmitted in any form or by any means. No transmission by electronic, mechanical including photocopying, digital, recorded or otherwise, without the prior written consent of the author or publisher.

This book and guide is based on discoveries made by researchers in the United States and Worldwide. It is rooted from the expertise of medical journals, scientific papers, medical reports, books, and other manuscripts.

This is NOT a free book or guide. So, you do not have the right to resell it.

Copyright 2019 © Healthy Kidney Publishing

ISBN: 978-0-9889442-4-4

Introduction

About the Author
My name is Robert Galarowicz ND, Naturopath and expert with advanced training in clinical & holistic nutrition.

I am like most people reading this book. I suffered with every stage of kidney disease from kidney failure, to the surgical creation of an A/V fistula, hemodialysis and am currently living with a kidney transplant that was received and still functions at stage 3 kidney disease.

Throughout this period, I began exploring and studying nutrition and holistic health which helped alleviate many of my problems. I began formal training in the nutrition and holistic health sciences, and after my kidney transplant I began private practice using the latest scientific research. I have worked with thousands of people personally and thousands more have purchased my products. With the feedback I get, and seeing before and after results, I know what works and what doesn't.

I use the same diets, supplements and life style recommendations for myself that I recommend to others to help improve your kidney disease. So, I personally understand the struggles anyone faces dealing with chronic kidney disease.

With the abundance of information and opinions available, there is contradictory information, and the field of kidney disease is no different. My advice is as long as the diet, supplement or lifestyle treatment is safe and has scientific credence you can always do a before and after lab work to see the results and make decisions from there.

Table of Contents

Page 1, Legal Disclaimer

Page 3, Introduction

Page 6, Which Diet Should You Choose

Page 11, Protein and Amino Acids When On A Low to Very Low Protein Diet

Page 18, The Low to Very Low Protein Diet

Page 24, The Low to Very Low Protein Diet Kidney Friendly Food List

Page 34, The Low to Very Low Protein Diet Plate Method

Page 35, The Low to Very Low Protein Diet Sample Menu Plan

Page 64, Essential Amino Acid Products & Companies

Page 67, Low Protein Food Companies

Page 69, The Vegetarian Diet for Kidney Disease Diet

Page 74, The Vegetarian Diet for Kidney Disease Food List

Page 86, The Vegetarian Diet for Kidney Disease Plate Method

Page 87, The Vegetarian Diet for Kidney Disease Sample Menu Plan

Page 118, The Academy of Nutrition and Dietetics Kidney Disease Diet

Page 122, The Academy of Nutrition and Dietetics Kidney Disease Diet Food List

Page 127, The Academy of Nutrition and Dietetics 'MyPlate' Method

Page 128, The Academy of Nutrition and Dietetics Sample Menu Plan

Page 158, Guides to Use With All 3 Dietary Approaches

Page 158, The Importance of Water and Hydration

Page 158, Eating Out With Kidney Disease

Page 160, Low Protein Eating Out Guide

Page 161, Vegetarian Eating Out Guide

Page 162, Academy of Nutrition and Dietetics Eating Out Guide

Page 165, Cooking Techniques to Lower Potassium

Page 166, Blanching To Reduce Sodium Content

Page 167, How to Read a Food Label

Page 170, Baking & Bread Making

Page 171, Final Thoughts

Which Diet Should You Choose?

This is the most common question and most important when it comes to anyone looking to improve his or her kidney disease. If you search the internet and speak to a variety of doctors and nutritional professionals, you will get conflicting and confusing information.

Many diets have been studied for a variety of kidney diseases. We have narrowed down the clinical research, along with my experience working with thousands of clients, to three diets that have shown consistent benefits in a variety of kidney diseases.

The three diets are:

- Low to Very Low Protein Diet Supplemented with Essential Amino Acids

- Vegetarian Diet For Kidney Disease

- Academy of Nutrition and Dietetics Kidney Disease Diet

Which diet you choose depends on a variety of factors we will cover. Such as the stage of your kidney disease and if you have diabetic kidney disease, medically termed, 'diabetic nephropathy.'

The second factor to take into account is what diet you will be able to stay on day in and day out every day of the year even through holidays, family gatherings, etc.

Another option is a combination of diets, which works for many people. An example of this is: someone may follow the low protein diet with essential amino acids, but on weekends with family events, eating out, etc., they will find The Academy of Nutrition and Dietetics kidney diet is more manageable.

Below we will get into the specifics of which diet is best for you. Regardless of whatever diet you choose, all will provide some degree of benefit. If you are unsure of what diet to choose, feel free to contact us and one of our health coaches will assist you.

Determining Your Ideal Diet Plan

Before you decide what diet is best suited for you a few questions need to be answered.

If your kidney disease is caused by diabetes or diabetic nephropathy, go to the section below titled, "Choosing The Proper Diet For Diabetic Nephropathy."

Do you have protein in your urine (proteinuria)?

Protein in the urine, medically termed proteinuria, is the biggest factor leading to the progression of kidney disease.

To find out if you have proteinuria, ask your medical doctor. This can be tested by a urine analysis, a 24-hour urine test or you can test at home using urinalysis reagent strips.

If you have protein in the urine, the ideal choice for you is the low to very low protein diet with supplemental amino acids. Your second option is the vegetarian diet for kidney disease.

These two diets have been shown to be the most effective at decreasing protein in the urine. If these two diets are not feasible for you, you can follow The Academy of Nutrition and Dietetics kidney disease diet. It is still very beneficial and can help lower protein in the urine.

Are you in stage 1 or stage 2 kidney disease?

If you are in stage 1 kidney disease, there is minimal damage and most likely no proteinuria. Therefore, The Academy of Nutrition and Dietetics kidney diet is suitable. If you would like a more aggressive approach, the vegetarian diet will suffice.

If you are in stage 2 kidney disease, you can most likely follow The Academy of Nutrition and Dietetics kidney diet. If you have proteinuria the better option is the vegetarian diet.

When stage 2 kidney disease is present, there is mild kidney damage and I would recommend an aggressive approach even in this earlier stage.

An aggressive approach taken at this point will provide very high chances of avoiding kidney failure for life. The vegetarian diet and the low protein diet with essential amino acids can be used.

Are you in stage 3a or 3b kidney disease?

If you are in stage 3a or 3b kidney disease, moderate to severe kidney damage is present.

The ideal diet is the low to very low protein diet followed by the vegetarian diet for kidney disease.

In stage 3b there is significant kidney damage and its better to follow a low to very low protein diet. This will provide the best chances of improving your kidney health and avoiding stage 4 kidney disease.
If you find either diet to be difficult to follow an option is the vegetarian diet with small amounts of animal protein from The Academy of Nutrition and Dietetics kidney diet.

Are you in stage 4 kidney disease?

If yes, the ideal diet shown to prevent kidney failure is the low to very low protein diet with supplemental amino acids. Your second option is the vegetarian diet for kidney disease. Its highly recommended to follow the very low protein diet with essential amino acids. This aggressive approach is recommended at this stage to avoid kidney failure.

Are you in stage 5 kidney disease?

If yes, the ideal diet is the very low protein diet with supplemental essential amino acids. At this stage, very little kidney function is present and if you're in the middle-to-end of stage 5, most likely dialysis can't be avoided. Make sure you're under proper care from a nephrologist.

Choosing The Proper Diet For Diabetic Nephropathy

When it comes to diabetic nephropathy, the ideal diet choice is not such a clear option. Balancing blood sugar with a therapeutic kidney diet can be problematic. What may work for one person may not work for another.

Below are some guidelines to follow. However, you know your body best and may need to alter foods and your diet based on your experience, carbohydrates and experimentation with new foods.

Are you in stage 1 or stage 2 Diabetic Nephropathy?

If yes, The Academy of Nutrition and Dietetics kidney diet is suitable. It will allow adequate blood sugar control. If you would like a more aggressive approach, the vegetarian diet will suffice.

If in stage 2, The Academy of Nutrition and Dietetics kidney diet with vegetarian sources of protein from the vegetarian diet is a good option. A more aggressive approach is the vegetarian diet.

Are you in stage 3a or 3b Diabetic Nephropathy?

If yes, continue to the next question.

Is your blood sugar and hemoglobin A1C under control?

If yes, the low to very low protein with essential amino acids or the vegetarian diet is ideal. It will most likely allow for adequate blood sugar control and reduce stress on the kidneys.

If no, the ideal diet is the Vegetarian Diet or the Vegetarian Diet with some animal sources of protein from The Academy of Nutrition and Dietetics.

If the vegetarian diet does not allow proper blood sugar control. Follow The Academy of Nutrition and Dietetics kidney diet.

Are you in stage 4 Diabetic Nephropathy?

If yes, the ideal diet shown to prevent diabetic kidney failure is the low to very low protein diet with supplemental amino acids. Your second option is the vegetarian diet for kidney disease.

The best option at this point is to limit proteins. Proteins will accelerate the loss of kidney function. Have plenty of fruits, and vegetables to keep blood sugar in control and consume the recommended supplements for blood sugar control listed in the main guide. Do this along with taking all your medications.

Are you in stage 5 Diabetic Nephropathy?

If yes, the ideal diet is the very low protein diet with supplemental essential amino acids. At this stage, very little kidney function is present and if you're in the middle-to-end of stage 5, most likely dialysis can't be avoided. Make sure you're under proper care from a nephrologist.

Protein and Amino Acids When On A Low To Very Low Protein Diet

The literature for low to very low protein diets for kidney disease dates back to a hundred years ago. It was even known back then that restricting protein can reverse, stop or slow down kidney disease.

The major problem is many people would become protein deficient, which leads to additional complications and risk of death in kidney disease.

This issue has been solved with the invention and application of supplemental essential amino acids for low to very low protein diets.

Essential amino acids are broken down proteins without any metabolic toxins from protein digestion that the kidney has to filter.

Essential amino acids also correct a problem seen in kidney disease called Protein Energy Malnutrition, which is covered in the main guide.

In the United States, essential amino acids are sold over the counter as nutritional supplements. Make sure to read the following section 'Essential Amino Acid Products & Companies' to see recommended brands to purchase and amounts to use.

Keto Analogues of Essential Amino Acids

Often called keto acids or keto analogues of essential amino acids. These are essential amino acids without nitrogen. Keto acids are more easily used by the body and are a better option than essential amino acids, because they contain no nitrogen. Nitrogen is a toxin your kidney will have to filter out.

However, these are typically expensive, costing $200 to $400 for a 4 week supply. Additionally, they are not easily available in the United States. They cause an increased risk of heart disease from high amounts of calcium used.

Essential Amino Acids are great for improving, stopping or slowing kidney disease with a low protein diet. Keto acids with a low protein diet are better, but due to cost and access, are not feasible for most people.

We listed two keto acid companies in the sections titled Essential Amino Acid Products & Companies.

Protein and Amino Acids

When digested, protein is broken down into *amino acids;* amino acids make up protein. There are twenty different amino acids used in building proteins. Of these 20 amino acids, 12 can be made by the body.

The other 8 cannot, we must consume them in our diet or through supplements.

These 12 amino acids are known as *non-essential* and the 8 are known as *essential*. Therefore, amino acids are divided into two categories, *essential and non-essential*.

Essential means that the body cannot produce the specific amino acid and they to be taken from outside sources, either through food or supplements.

Non-essential amino acids can be made by the body, but can also be obtained from the diet.

The low to very low protein diet begins to show benefit when the protein consumption starts at (0.6 grams protein x body weight in kilograms (kg) per day) all the way down to a very low protein diet (0.3 grams protein x body weight in kilograms (kg) per day).

Studies show for every 0.2 grams of protein reduction x kilogram of body weight can result in a 29% slower rate of loss of kidney function and, in some cases, stop progression of kidney disease.

The amount of protein you decide to consume will be based on your ability to follow a low or very low protein diet. For best results you should be consuming (0.3 grams protein x body weight in kilograms [kg] per day), but excellent results have been shown up to the (0.6 grams protein x body weight in kilograms [kg] per day) as long as you don't go over 40 to 45 grams of protein per day.

You will need to decide what amount of protein consumption fits your lifestyle and dietary habits.

However, stay between 0.3 and 0.6 grams of protein x body weight in kilograms per day. You should be consuming no more than 40 to 45 grams of protein per day, regardless of the sum of your calculations.

Remember, the closer you are to 0.3 grams of protein per day, the greater the benefits.

Note: When you drop below 0.6 grams of protein you will need some form of essential amino acids to avoid protein deficiency. This will be explained in the following pages.

Now, let's figure out how much protein you should be consuming.

Calculating Protein Consumption

To benefit from this diet you will need to calculate how much protein you need to consume.

First, determine your weight in kilograms. Divide your body weight by 2.2 which is 1 kilogram (kg). 1 pound = 2.2 kilograms.

You can now decide how much protein you need each day by multiplying your body weight in kilograms by 0.3, 0.4, 0.5, 0.6.

Example: 175 pounds divided by 2.2 gives us the weight in kilograms of 79.

If you were following the very low protein diet you will multiply 79 x 0.3 which results in 23 to 24 grams of protein per day.

If you find consuming very low protein (0.3 grams of protein which equals about 21 to 25 grams per day) will not work for you, then multiply your body weight by 0.4, 0.5 or 0.6 grams of protein for higher amounts.

However, do not go over 40 to 45 grams of protein per day if kidney disease is present. Remember, even if your calculation is above 40 to 45 grams per day you still should not exceed 40 to 45 grams per day.

Note: Often in life social events, food cravings, etc., will have us go over our daily protein count. This can be frustrating and lead to us stopping everything. A positive outlook should always be maintained. Even if amounts of protein are over 45 grams per day, by minimizing the protein (any amount) will improve your kidney health. If you have a bad meal or snack, forgive yourself, leave the emotions in the past, and move on, remaining focused on your diet for the next meal or snack.

Sample Protein Calculations

- 175lbs divided by 2.2 kilos = 79 x 0.3 = 23 grams of protein per day

- 175lbs divided by 2.2 kilos = 79 x 0.4 = 31 grams of protein per day

- 175lbs divided by 2.2 kilos = 79 x 0.5 = 39 grams of protein per day

- 175lbs divided by 2.2 kilos = 79 x 0.6 = 47 grams of protein per day

How to Count Protein in Foods

Many of the foods we consume will have some degree of protein in them. This will vary from very small amounts, such as an apple, to large amounts found in animal sources (meat, fish, eggs, dairy). You will need to track your protein intake from foods to stay within your guidelines.

Most food labels will have the protein count in them. If you don't know how to read a food label that is covered in its own section.

Essential Amino Acids & Malnutrition

As mentioned earlier, when on the low or very low protein diet, you will require essential amino acid supplementation to avoid protein deficiency.

The 8 essential amino acids need to be consumed from supplemental sources in order to keep an adequate nutritional balance.

One amino acid called L-Histidine is considered a semi-essential amino acid because adults generally produce adequate amounts but children may not. However, in kidney disease, it is believed the body lacks the ability to produce histidine, therefore it will need to be consumed along with the 8 essential amino acids.

The 8 essential amino acids are:

Isoleucine	L-Leucine	L-Lysine
L-Methionine	L-Phenylalanine	L-Threonine
L-Tryptophan	L-Valine	

You will need to consume anywhere from 3.0 to 4.0 grams (3000-4000 mg) of essential amino acids and histidine once to three times per day with meals. With most commercial essential amino acid products available, this will come out to 3 to 6 pills once to three times per day with meals. The mixture of amino acids can also be taken as a powder.

In many cases, you can consume less pills and powders depending on your protein consumption and albumin blood work numbers which is discussed on the following pages.

Here is a list of each milligram dose of essential amino acids and l-histidine required one to three times per day to avoid protein malnutrition

If you are close to the amounts listed you will be ok and avoid protein malnutrition.

L-Isoleucine 400 mg	L-Leucine 600 mg	L-Lysine 400 mg
L-Methionine 600 mg	L-Phenylalanine 600 mg	L-Threonine 300 mg
L-Tryptophan 150 mg	L-Valine 500 mg	L-Histidine 300 mg

If you purchase one of the recommended brands they will be dosed properly, therefore no calculations of amino acids are needed.

There have also been many people who have purchased essential amino acids individually and in combined quantities and have been able to make up the recommended amounts.

For example, you can use an L-lysine pill that is 500mg per day three times per day to meet your daily protein nutritional need of that amino acid. You can also use BCAA (Branch Chained Amino Acids) pills or powders which are made up of L-Leucine, L-Isoleucine, and L-Valine to meet amino acid nutritional needs.

There are also mixtures of the essential amino acids, in smaller doses, along with other non-essential amino acids in pill and powder forms readily available. This can be combined with essential amino acids to prevent protein malnutrition, but since smaller doses are used, you will need to consume larger amounts of pills and powders.

Depending on your access to essential amino acids there are many options available to prevent protein malnutrition and help your kidneys. Ideally, you should strive to use only the essential amino acids and not the non-essential amino acids, as this approach has shown the most benefit in kidney disease.

Monitoring Blood Work for Protein Energy Malnutrition

There is a blood test called albumin, which is the major protein of blood; albumin (the same name as the test) plays an important role in maintaining fluid balance (osmotic pressure) inside blood vessels, in transporting drugs, hormones, and enzymes, and used to determine protein malnutrition.

When low albumin levels are seen in kidney disease, albumin is leaking from the blood into the urine and being lost. This is known as proteinuria.

This blood test range is from 3.5 to 5.5 g/dl. For optimal status you will want to keep your albumin 4.0 g/dl or higher. Dropping under 4.0 g/dl is considered protein deficiency and poorer outcomes in CKD are seen.

If you are below 4.0 g/dl an increase in essential amino acids is needed. If your blood test albumin count is 4.5 g/dl or greater you can consume fewer essential amino acid supplements, but you don't have to.

Being above 4.0 g/dl is completely fine. However, if you find consuming the essential amino supplements difficult and you are above 4.5 g/dl you can reduce the amounts, but make sure to be 4.0 g/dl or greater.

The Low To Very Low Protein Diet™

This is a 2-week diet plan, including recipes and tips for eating out. Most recipes will serve 4 people.

You can mix and match the meal plans to your liking and don't have to consume as many snacks as listed. You should be taking some form of essential amino acids with meals or snacks.

Each day of the diet will fluctuate between 22 grams to a maximum of 45 grams per day of protein.

When food shopping, choose the lowest protein, potassium and salt products available.

Making your own meals and snacks

There are many more menu and snack options available aside from what is included in this guide. When making your own dishes you can modify other recipes by taking out protein foods such as dairy, eggs, beans, nuts, seeds, soy, etc., and replacing with rice or almond milk, oils and small amounts of starches and flour.

Also, many vegan recipes only need to be slightly modified by eliminating the protein foods and cutting down on amounts of vegetables and fruits, if you need to reduce potassium.

Overview of Diet

Dietary management of kidney disease is not to be underestimated. Diet is the most important factor in preserving and improving the kidneys. Without a therapeutic diet, most efforts to preserve and improve your kidneys will have little long-term effect.

This low to very low protein diet has an interesting history, and a scientific theory that gives it credence. Review it and give it careful consideration.

The Diet You Should Be Following

Consuming a low or very low protein diet along with low phosphorus, low to moderate potassium, low sodium, higher alkaline, high fiber has shown to have excellent results in improving, stopping or slowing down diabetic kidney disease.

Did I create this diet? Partially. The "core" of this low to very low protein diet has been known for 100 years as a treatment for chronic kidney disease, but I made modifications to it which provide additional benefits.

The "base" of this low to very low protein diet with supplemental amino acids, has been used for the last 35 years with great success in the Czech Republic, Hungary, Brazil, Italy, Mexico, China, France, Mideast, etc.

It became popularized in the United States from a book called "Coping with Kidney Disease: A 12-Step Treatment Program to Help You Avoid Dialysis," by Mackenzie Walser MD & Betsy Thorpe.

Let's get started.

I will briefly touch upon each part of the diet, so you will have a good understanding of how it will help chronic kidney disease.

Low or Very Low Protein

Dietary protein intake results in a faster rate of declining kidney function. This is because protein results in the accumulation of nitrogen waste products, urea, hydrogen ions, phosphates, and inorganic ions which have to be eliminated or regulated by the kidney. Dietary protein lost during kidney disease (proteinuria) has also been shown to create inflammation further damaging the kidney.

Healthy kidneys can handle normal to large amounts of dietary protein, and keep the body in balance. When kidney disease is present, filtering out these waste products puts an increased stress on the kidneys leading to eventual loss of function.

Consuming a low or very low protein diet takes the stress of performing these functions off of the kidney leading to improving, slowing or arresting the kidney disease. It also improves nutritional status, with essential amino acid supplementation, and improves symptoms of kidney disease including uremia.

Uremia is a clinical syndrome associated with fluid, toxin buildup, electrolyte, and hormone imbalances and metabolic abnormalities which develop in parallel with loss of renal function.

Eating very low or low protein is the most important part of this diet. The diet and research recommend consuming 22 to 26 grams of protein per day for best results, but great success has been achieved with higher amounts of protein of up to 45 grams per day maximum. This protein amount can be adjusted depending on your needs, wants and lifestyle with no ill effects.

For example, on Monday you have 25 grams of protein and Tuesday you have 40 grams and Wednesday 30 grams, Thursday 22, Friday 25, etc.

Take a moment to think of your kidney like a car engine. If you make a car engine work harder by driving it a lot, eventually the engine will stop working after a certain number of miles. This same concept applies to your kidneys, especially when kidney damage is present. The more it has to work eliminating protein waste products and continuously controlling body functions the faster you will lose kidney function.

Attention: When the diet contains less than the minimum amount of 0.6 grams of protein per kilogram of body weight per day (0.6 g protein x kilogram (kg) b.w./day), it is crucial to supplement the diet with essential amino acids or the pharmaceutical brand (ketosterils/ketoacids, not available in U.S.) to meet the nutritional needs of the body.

Without taking these amino acids on the low to very low protein diet, you are bound to develop protein deficiency.

Components of The Diet

Low Phosphorus

Phosphorus is another important mineral that the kidneys need to keep regulated. In kidney disease, phosphorus levels can become elevated leading to complications with the skeletal system (bones), the body's energy production, and cell functioning. High levels also put more stress on the kidneys, forcing them to work harder which leads to a faster decline in function. Luckily, most absorbable phosphorus is contained in protein rich foods.

Low to Moderate Potassium

Potassium is one of the main minerals of the body. It plays a critical role in heart functioning through muscular contraction. The kidneys are responsible for excreting 90% of the potassium from the body. In diabetic kidney disease, there may be either too little potassium or too much (too much is known as hyperkalemia). It's much more common to have hyperkalemia in kidney disease.

Hyperkalemia can lead to dysrhythmias (irregular heartbeats) and cardiac arrest. This along with high potassium levels may cause further damage to the kidneys. This is why a low to moderate potassium diet is being suggested.

You may think *why not consume a low potassium diet*? In order to maintain low protein consumption -- the most important part -- you have to consume moderate amounts of potassium foods to maintain good nutritional status.

Low Sodium

Sodium is essential for many body functions including regulating the blood pressure and blood volume, helping transmit impulses for nerve function, muscle contractions and regulating the acid-alkaline (*aka* acid-base) balance of blood and body fluids.

When kidney disease is present, extra sodium can build up in the body leading to fluid accumulation. This can cause swollen ankles, puffiness, a rise in blood pressure, shortness of breath, and/or fluid around your heart and lungs which can lead to heart failure. Keeping sodium levels low is important to maintaining overall health with kidney disease. Salt should never be added to foods. Don't purchase food with high amounts of salt. Ideally, sodium intake should not exceed 2000mg per day. Its best to stay at 1500mg or less per day.

Higher Alkaline

The kidneys maintain the acid-alkaline balance of the body (Ph level). When too much acid builds up in the body from acidic foods and the kidneys cannot keep the balance, the results are inflammation, chronic illness and worsening of kidney function.

This is why a higher alkaline diet is preferred. Every food is either considered alkaline or acidic, and maintaining a higher amount of alkaline foods will help take the stress off your kidneys. Fresh fruits and vegetables like cauliflower, lettuce, onions, peas, peppers, apples, berries, grapes and lemons are quick and effective ways to incorporate more alkaline foods into your diet.

High Fiber

A high fiber diet of 20 to 35 grams per day from food and supplements has shown to slow and improve kidney disease. Fiber has anti-inflammatory benefits and clears toxins out of the gastrointestinal tract, which build up in kidney disease. In order to achieve a high fiber diet without the additional potassium from fruits and vegetables, a supplement may be introduced.

Vegetarian

Why vegetarian? All animal sources of food (dairy, eggs, chicken, meats including beef, lamb, goat, etc.) have been shown to decrease kidney function once there is damage. The reason is that after digestion of animal proteins, more urea and toxins need to be filtered by your kidneys. Vegetarian food sources have been shown to delay kidney function and nutrients like phosphorus aren't easily absorbed from vegetarian sources of food.

Anti-Inflammatory & Anti-Oxidant

This diet will have many healthy, good anti-inflammatory fats and other foods, which have been shown to help kidney disease. For example, sesame oil has been shown to help protect and help injured kidneys recover because of the anti-inflammatory and anti-oxidant benefits and ability to help control the body's glucose level. Glucose level is the amount of glucose (*aka* "sugar or blood sugar") within the body. When the body's glucose remains high, this can lead to further kidney damage.

Anti-inflammatory and anti-oxidant foods are important for those major reasons. Many fruits in the berry family, such as strawberries, blueberries and cherries, have been shown to significantly reduce inflammation, along with being renowned for their anti-oxidant properties. Another great anti-inflammatory agent is olive oil, so be sure to use it in your foods whenever you can. And, in addition to its kidney-boosting ability, it should come as no surprise that green tea is another rich source of anti-inflammatory/anti-oxidant properties.

The Low to Very Low Protein Kidney Friendly Food List

The below foods are considered very kidney friendly. They are low in potassium, phosphorus, protein and some have therapeutic value such as anti-inflammatory and anti-oxidant benefits to combat kidney damage.

Frozen, Fresh and Canned Foods
It is best to use fresh or frozen foods because of the lower salt content of fresh foods and, in most cases, lower potassium content of frozen foods compared to canned foods. Typically, the higher sodium content of frozen and canned foods, and the added sugar often makes them undesirable. If you can, find frozen and canned foods without salt and added sugar.

Fats and Oils

Any oils can be used but the following have shown special benefits

Sesame seed oil and flax seed oil
These two oils have shown the most benefit, aside from fish oil, when kidney disease is present. You should avoid cooking with flax seed oil, as it can become a source of free radicals when heated.

Canola, coconut and walnut oil
These three oils have shown benefit in kidney disease.

Extra virgin olive oil
This oil has shown healthy benefits to your cardiac and vascular system.

Butter
Butter has not been shown to be either harmful or beneficial to

the kidneys. Consider it neutral, so small amounts are acceptable. However, butter and mayo should be your last choice for fats and should be avoided if there is high cholesterol.

Vinegars, Salt, Seasonings and Condiments

Vinegars
All vinegars are acceptable with kidney disease; make sure no salt is added.

Salt, Seasonings and Condiments
Avoid table salt and any seasonings that have the word "salt or sodium," and avoid salt substitutes (they contain potassium) and any seasonings with potassium. Purchase the lowest sodium foods you can and don't add salt to any foods. Most other seasonings are acceptable. Keep sodium intake to 1500-2000mg per day.

List of Seasonings and Condiments
Allspice, basil, bay leaf, caraway seed, chives, cilantro, cinnamon, cloves, cumin, curry, dill, extracts (almond, lemon, lime, maple, orange, peppermint, vanilla, walnut), fennel, garlic powder, ginger, horseradish (root), lemon juice, low sodium hot sauce like Tabasco®, mustard, Mrs. Dash®, nutmeg, onion powder or flakes, oregano, paprika, parsley flakes, pepper (ground), pimentos, poppy seed, rosemary, saffron, sage, savory, sesame seeds, tarragon, thyme, turmeric, vegan mayo (not made with soy, check protein content).

Salad Dressings
It is best to make your own with oil, vinegar, spices and, vegan mayo. Some Russian, French, and Ranch dressings have low potassium and protein levels and can be consumed.

Jelly, Jams and Honey

Jelly, Jams and Honey
These are simple sugars that contain only small amounts of potassium, sodium or phosphorus when used in the amounts listed to consume. You can have between two to five tablespoons per day. It is best to stay to near two tablespoons and look for the least amount of sugar when purchasing jams and jellies.

Beverages

Water, Green Tea, Hibiscus Tea
Consume more of your beverages from water, green and hibiscus tea. You can consume 2-3 cups (16-24 ounces) of tea per day. Consuming green and hibiscus tea has shown to benefit the kidneys.

Chamomile and Black Tea
If you find you do not like green tea or hibiscus tea, you can substitute with 16-24 ounces per day of chamomile and black tea. They have some benefit for kidney disease, but not as much as green tea. Chamomile should be your first choice and black tea the second.

A Word about Teas
In the early stages of kidney disease (1, 2 and most likely all of stage 3) you can consume higher amounts of teas, but make sure you have your potassium checked before and after doing this. There are no restrictions on teas. Any teas are ok to consume with kidney disease.

Rice and Almond Milk
Rice milk and almond milk can be consumed because they are low in potassium, phosphorus and protein. It can be used as a replacement for milk in cooking or baking. Flavored varieties are available which have a little more potassium and phosphorus than non-flavored.

Fruits

Apple	Apple Sauce	Apple Butter
Apples, Dried	Blackberries	Blueberries
Cherries	Cranberries	Dried Cranberries
Grapes	Lemon	Lime
Pineapple	Plums	Raspberries
Strawberries	Tangerines	

Vegetables

Alfalfa Seeds, Sprouted Raw	Asparagus	Bean Sprouts
Cabbage	Corn	Cauliflower
Green Beans	Eggplant	Jicama
Leeks	Lettuce, all kinds	Mushrooms, shiitake
Onions	Peas, Green	Peppers, chili
Scallions	Radicchio	Radishes

Breads/Cereals/Grains - Find the Lowest Salt, Sugar and Lowest Protein Products Made Up of the Grains Below

Whole Grains

Whole grains have higher amounts of phosphorus and potassium and should be avoided or limited in the later stages of kidney disease. Choose refined grains, which are usually listed on the package label as refined, enriched, or the grain doesn't have the word "whole" before it. For example, whole wheat may be listed or just wheat. Whole wheat is the whole grain and if wheat is just listed that is the refined grain.

However, in stages 1, 2, and 3 of kidney disease you can have more whole grains in your diet, provided your phosphorus and potassium levels are in mid-range.

Make Sure to Choose the Lowest Protein and Unsalted

Or the lowest sodium products you can find for all foods listed. Remember to read all labels and check all products.

Bread, Cereals and Grain Products

Wheat Flour	Bagels	Bread Sticks
Bulgur Wheat	Couscous	Crackers, Wheat
Croissants	Dinner Rolls or Hard Rolls	English Muffins
French Bread	Italian Bread	Light Rye
Melba Toast	Noodles	Oyster Crackers
Pancakes	Pasta, all kinds	Pita bread
Pretzels	Soft Wheat	Tortillas
Waffles	White/Wheat Bread	

Corn

Corn Flour/Meal	Corn Chips (unsalted)	Corn Grits
Corn Muffins	Corn Tortillas	Corn Pancakes, made with no eggs
Popcorn (unsalted)		

Rice

Rice Flour	Most White Rices	Rice Pasta
Rice Bread	Rice Cakes	Rice Crackers
Cassava, aka Tapioca or Yuca	Tapioca Flour/Starch, not the root vegetable	

Cassava, aka Tapioca or Yuca & Potato

Tapioca Flour/Starch, not the root vegetable
Potato Flour/Starch

Gluten Free Products

Some gluten free products are acceptable depending on the flour source used. Check protein content, sodium and if labeled potassium.

Breads	Pancakes
Waffles	Crackers

Cereals, Dry

Corn Flakes	Puffed Wheat
Rice Cereal	Other cereals with crisp, chex or puff in the name

Cereals, Hot

Cream of Rice	Cream of Wheat	Grits
Malt-O-Meal	Wheat Farina	For more flavor, consider cinnamon, kidney friendly fruit or Tabasco® (a favorite for grits).

Soup Broths

Use a base of water or low potassium, low protein, low salt commercial brands and avoid drinking the broth.

Going Very Low Protein

If you decide to go very low protein (20 to 25 grams per day) in your diet, you may need to purchase specialty products and very low protein flours for baking. You can eat very low protein provided you have access to many different food varieties, which are usually found in major cities or areas with dense populations.

For those who don't have easy access to large food varieties, I included a list of specialty low protein companies on page 111 which lists companies that offer these products and resources.

Moderately Kidney-Friendly Foods and Beverages Juices

8 ounces (1 cup) of juices or below have acceptable amounts of potassium (100-150mg).	Be mindful to not have too much juice in your diet as the potassium content can rise quickly. No more than 4 to 8 ounces per day.	Cranberry juice
Grape juice bottled - 6 ounces maximum	Grape juice Frozen	Crangrape Juice
Cranapple Juice	Lemonade	Pear nectar

Sweeteners

Maple syrup

Natural Sweeteners

Stevia, aka Stevia Rebaudiana (Truvia™, PureVia™) is a zero calorie natural sweetener taken from herbaceous perennial plant from the genus Stevia Cav. Rebaudioside A and stevioside are steviol glycosides which are extracts taken from the leaves that have been used as natural sweeteners for over 25 years in South America, Brazil and Japan. It has a Generally Recognized as Safe (GRAS) status as a general-purpose sweetener for food and drink by the FDA.

Research has shown benefits when diabetes, hypertension and kidney disease is present. Moderate amounts can be consumed, even in baking, until more is known.

Condiments

Mayonnaise, 1-2 tbsp. per day

Fruits

Elderberries	Olives, (blanched)	Orange
Peaches	Pears	Honeydew
Watermelon		

Vegetables

Beets	Broccoli	Brussels sprouts
Carrots	Celery	Collards
Mushrooms	Okra	Potato Chips
Squash	Sweet Potato	

Unfriendly Kidney Foods List

Beverages

Fruit Juices, Soft Drinks, Coffee
Other fruit juices, not listed in kidney friendly foods and sodas/soft drinks should be avoided due to fructose (fruit sugar) intake, higher potassium and phosphorus levels. Fructose and sugar (mentioned below) added to soft drinks such as soda, ginger ale, etc., and other fruit juices have been shown to create inflammation, contribute to high blood pressure, obesity, diabetes and increase the risk of further damage to the kidneys.

Coffee
Coffee should be limited to 1, 8oz cup per day. We once believed coffee is bad for kidney disease. Recent research possibly shows a benefit. Further studies need to be conducted before a definitive answer is known.

Alcohol
Alcohol consumption should be avoided in CKD. If you want to have alcohol, red wine is preferred for kidney disease.

Sweeteners and Artificial Sweeteners

Sugar/Sucrose
Sugar, *aka* sucrose, should be minimized or eliminated in kidney disease. Sugar is very difficult to avoid as it's added to many products including breads. Small amounts are acceptable within the diet, but large amounts should be avoided by eliminating sugary beverages and large amounts of baked goods, cookies, cakes, pies, candies, etc.

High sugar/sucrose intake has been shown to increase the risk of diabetes, worsen its condition, suppress the immune system, increase uric acid, decrease HDL (good) cholesterol, and cause digestive symptoms such as gas, bloating, and diarrhea.

Fructose and High-Fructose Corn Syrup
Fructose, a popular ingredient in beverages, and HFCS should be minimized or avoided, as the problems associated with sucrose and fructose apply to high fructose corn syrup as well.

Sugar Alcohols
Sugar alcohols such as sorbitol, erythritol, xylitol, mannitol, lactitol and maltitol. Not much is known about these sweeteners and their connection to kidney disease. Small amounts in combination with Stevia can be consumed, but they should be limited until further research is conducted.

Artificial Sweeteners
Avoid all artificial sweeteners as some have been shown to be harmful to the nervous system and brain. They can raise the risk of cancer, and there is concern over their involvement in other health problems. Many artificial sweeteners have not been studied in relation to kidney disease and should be avoided until further research is conducted.

Here is a list of artificial sweeteners: Saccharin (Sweet'N Low®, SugarTwin®), Aspartame (NutraSweet®, Equal®), Acesulfame K (ACK, Sunett®, Sweet One®), Sucralose (Splenda®), and the recent Neotame.

Fruits and Vegetables

Avoid the exotic star fruit, as it has shown to be very toxic to the kidney. Other fruits, vegetables, as well as friendly and moderately-friendly kidney foods may be consumed in liberal quantities if your blood tests show your potassium levels are in range. The issue with these foods is the potassium content. If you need strict control over your potassium levels then the fruits and vegetables not listed should be avoided.

Low To Very Low Protein Diet Plate Method
Use this as a guide for choosing portion size and balancing nutrients

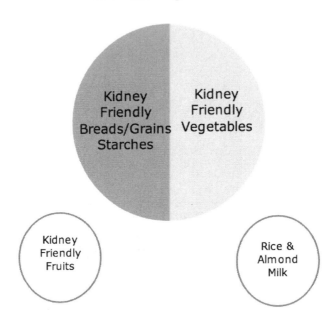

Additional Beverages: Kidney Friendly Teas & Juices.

The Low to Very Low Protein Sample Menu Plan

Week 1, Day 1

Breakfast
2 cups rice cereal
1 to 2 cups rice milk
1 cup blueberries
1 apple

Lunch
Low Protein Sandwich
Apple – 1 small to moderate size

Snack
2 cups popcorn

Dinner
1 to 2 cups *Spicy Gold Rice*
You can add 2 to 3 tablespoons of kidney-friendly oil to any rice dish

Snack
10 corn chips
½ cup grapes

Nutrition Content For Day
Calories: 1,524
Fat: 32 g, 9 g saturated
Protein: 31.6 g
Potassium: 629 mg
Phosphorus: 293 mg

Recipes For The Day
Low Protein Sandwich
Ingredients:
2 slices bread
1 tbsp oil/vinegar spread
1 slice eggplant
1 to 2 tomato slices
1 slice roasted pepper
1 to 2 slices of salad leaves

Directions:
Toast bread and spread oil/vinegar, layer on eggplant, tomato slices, roasted pepper and salad leaves.

Spicy Gold Rice
Ingredients:
2 ½ tbsp. sesame oil
1 small onion, chopped
1 medium jalapeno pepper, minced
½ tsp. ground turmeric
¼ tsp. ground cinnamon
1 cup long grain rice
water for rice
1 bay leaf

Directions:
In a saucepan, heat oil over medium low heat. Add the onion, pepper and stir until onion is translucent, about 6 to 8 minutes.

Mix in turmeric and cinnamon. Add the rice and stir for 2 minutes to coat the rice with the spice mix. Add water, bring to boil, reduce heat to low, cover and cook until all liquid is absorbed.

Week 1, Day 2
Breakfast
2 waffles
2 tablespoon butter
1 ½ tablespoon jam

Snack
10 *Apple Rings*
1 cup rice milk

Lunch
1 to 1 ½ cup *Sunny Penne*
1 slice bread with ½ to 1 tablespoon butter

Snack
1 small plum
6 crackers

Dinner
1 to 2 cups *Spicy Gold Rice*
You can add 2 to 3 tablespoons of kidney-friendly oil to any rice dish

Nutrition Content For Day
Calories: 1,384
Fat: 58.5 g, 26 g saturated
Protein: 23.8 g
Potassium: 808 mg
Phosphorus: 314 mg

Recipes For The Day
Oven Dried Apples
Ingredients:
Apples, as many as desired
A few tbsp. fresh lemon juice
A pinch or two of Stevia (optional)

Directions:
Preheat the oven to 150 degrees. Core the apples and slice them into ½ inch rings. Soak in a bowl of water with the lemon juice for 15 minutes, and add the stevia if using. Drain, and lay in a single layer on top of cooling racks positioned on top of a baking sheet.

Place in the oven and bake for a couple of hours, depending really on whether you want crispy apple chips or chewy dried apples. You may want to flip the rings every now and then to cook them evenly, and keep in mind to check them individually as some of them may be done before others.

Sunny Penne
Ingredients:
3 medium carrots, peeled and thinly sliced
4 small zucchini, thinly sliced
¼ cup snap peas
2 medium plum tomatoes diced
½ small onion, sliced thin
1 red bell pepper, sliced thin
2 medium garlic cloves

1 tbsp. dried tarragon
4 tbsp. olive oil, sesame oil or walnut oil
1 tsp. white wine vinegar
12 oz. of dry penne pasta

Directions:
Bring medium saucepan of water to a boil. Put carrots and zucchini in the water for 2 minutes. Add the peas and cook for 1 minute longer. Drain well, place in a large bowl and add the tomatoes, pepper, onion, garlic, tarragon, oil, vinegar.

Cook pasta according to package direction. Drain when cooked, and top with sauce.

Week 1, Day 3
Breakfast
1 to 3 *Cornmeal Pancakes*
You can add 1 to 1 ½ tablespoons butter
1 to 2 tablespoons maple syrup

Lunch
1 ½ cup *Tomato Salad with Basil Vinaigrette*
1 to 2 tablespoons *Basil Vinaigrette*
1 small roll with *Savory Olive Oil*

Snack
1 cup pineapple
¾ cup corn Chex
¼ to ½ cup rice milk

Dinner
2 cups *Quick Pasta with Broccoli*

Snack
1 cup blueberries

Nutrition Content For Day
Calories: 1,936
Fat: 76.8 g, 26.1 g saturated
Protein: 32.7 g
Potassium: 871 mg
Phosphorus: 223 mg

Recipes For The Day
Cornmeal Pancakes
Ingredients:
1 1/2 cup vanilla rice milk
1/2 tsp. lemon juice
2 tbsp. sesame oil
1 1/3 cup all-purpose flour
1/2 cup coarse cornmeal
1 tsp. baking powder
1/2 tsp. baking soda
1 tsp. vanilla extract

Directions:
In a small mixing bowl, whisk together the rice milk, lemon juice and sesame oil, set aside. In another mixing bowl, sift together the remaining ingredients. Add the wet ingredients to the dry, mixing until just combined (avoid over mixing).

Heat a lightly oiled skillet or non-stick skillet over medium heat. Add the batter to the pan 1/4 cup at a time, cooking until the edges and surface are bubbly and the underside is golden brown. Using a spatula, flip the pancake and cook for about 1 minute more until both sides are golden brown. Repeat with remaining batter and serve hot with syrup.

Tomato Salad with Basil Vinaigrette
Ingredients:
4 cup red leaf lettuce
1 lb. vine-ripened tomatoes, cut into thick slices
½ pint cherry tomatoes
10 low sodium blanched olives, cut in half

Directions:
Chop lettuce in small sizes. Spread lettuce on a serving platter and arrange the sliced on top. Add cherry tomatoes and olives over salad. Drizzle with vinaigrette.

Basil Vinaigrette
Ingredients:
1 tbsp. champagne vinegar
¼ cup walnut oil

¼ cup packed basil leaves, coarsely chopped

Directions:
Combine all ingredients in a blender or small food processor. Blend until smooth.

Savory Olive Oil
Ingredients:
1 cup extra virgin olive oil
1 large garlic, cut in half
½ tsp. of minced herbs

Quick Pasta with Broccoli
Ingredients:
2 cup small broccoli florets
½ cup butter
2 tbsp. dried basil
2 tbsp. dried parsley
1 small clove garlic, minced
8 oz. of dry pasta of choice

Directions:
Cut broccoli tops into small florets. In a bowl combine butter, basil, parsley, garlicup Mix ingredients well. In a saucepan, bring 4 cups of water to a boil. Add the broccoli to boiling water and cook until tender. Drain and place in a bowl, add herb butter and toss coating the broccoli.

Cook pasta according to package directions. Drain well when cooked and top with broccoli and herb butter.

Week 1, Day 4
Breakfast
2 cups Cream of Wheat hot cereal, made with water
10 cherries

Snack
1 peach
1 cup popcorn

Lunch
2 cups *Chinese Noodle Salad*

Snack
1 cup jicama with low protein dipping sauce such as salad dressings.

Dinner
2 *Asian Vegetable Wraps*

Nutrition Content For Day
Calories: 1,705
Fat: 73.4 g, 9.1 g saturated
Protein: 29.2 g
Potassium: 1,402 mg
Phosphorus: 260 mg

Recipes For The Day
Chinese Noodle Salad
Ingredients:
1 garlic clove
1 inch piece of fresh ginger, peeled and sliced
1 tbsp. Kikkoman™ light soy sauce
2 tbsp. rice vinegar
¼ cup sesame oil
2 tbsp. olive oil
1 tsp. dried hot pepper seeds (crushed red pepper flakes)
1 medium red bell pepper, cut into ½ inch
¾ cup chopped green or white onions
3 ¼ cup cooked pasta of choice

Directions:
Process the garlic and ginger in a food processor until finely minced. Add the soy sauce, vinegar and blend. Add the two oils, hot pepper seeds and blend.

In a large bowl combine the dressing, pepper, and onions. Combine cooked pasta with vegetables and dressing. Serve warm or at room temperature.

Asian Vegetable Wraps
Ingredients:
2 tbsp. orange juice
3 tbsp. Kikkoman light soy sauce
2 tbsp. honey
1 pinch red pepper flakes (crushed red pepper flakes)
½ tsp. cornstarch
2 tbsp. of canola oil
1 small onion, cut in half and thinly sliced
2 medium stalks celery, cut in half and thinly sliced
1 small carrot, peeled and cut into matchsticks
1 medium zucchini, cut in half and into matchsticks
1 cup cooked rice of choice
8 corn tortillas

Directions:
Combine the orange juice, soy sauce, honey, cornstarch, and red pepper flakes in a small bowl. Stir well and set aside. In a large skillet, heat the oil over medium high heat until the oil is hot. Add the onion, celery, carrot and stir fry for another 3 minutes. Stir the soy sauce combination to remix and quickly add it to the vegetables, stirring constantly. The sauce should thicken and coat the vegetables. If it doesn't thicken, increase the heat a bit.

Add cooked rice to the vegetables and stir until heated through. Warm corn tortillas in oven or microwave, fill with Asian vegetable filling, and roll tortillas around filling.

Week 1, Day 5
Breakfast
4 ounces of yogurt such as Activia™ brand
1 slice of bread with jam or butter
1 tangerine

Lunch
1 ½ cups *Southern Pumpkin Soup* (Do not drink broths of any soups)**
8-10 crackers

Snack
1 apple

1 rice cake

Dinner
2 servings of *Boiled Potatoes and Vegetable Combo*

Snack
3 cups popcorn

Nutrition Content For Day
Calories: 1,166
Fat: 16.4 g, 3.7 g saturated
Protein: 27.1 g
Potassium: 2,542 mg
Phosphorus: 343 mg

Recipes For The Day
Southern Pumpkin Soup
Ingredients:
2 cup water
1 cup vegetable broth
1 cup liquid non-diary creamer
1 15-oz. can pumpkin
1 tbsp. brown sugar
1 tbsp. ground cumin
1 tsp. ground coriander
½ to 1 tsp. chili powder
You can add ½ cup croutons

Directions:
In a medium saucepan or stockpot, bring broth, water and non-dairy creamer to a boil over medium high heat. Mix in pumpkin, sugar, and spices.

Reduce heat to medium to low and simmer uncovered until soup thickens a little and flavors have blended, about 10 minutes. Season with pepper and serve with croutons if desired.

Boiled Potatoes and Vegetable Combo
Ingredients:
2 medium size potatoes, cut into large pieces
½ cup asparagus
½ cup sliced green beans

½ cup cauliflower flowerets

Directions:
Double-cook potatoes and put into fresh container. Add water to half full or enough to completely cover potatoes. Place metal strainer or steamer platform over potatoes and add the rest of the vegetables. Cover and heat to boiling, adjusting heat as necessary to prevent overflow. A moderate amount of steam should escape lid.

Cook 15-20 minutes or until potatoes and vegetables are soft. Pour remaining water off the potatoes. Combine potatoes and vegetables or leave separate. Season to taste.

Week 1, Day 6
Breakfast
Low Protein Shake
1 roll with butter
¾ cup watermelon

Lunch
1 to 1 ½ cups of *Boiled Vegetables* over
1 to 2 cups of rice

Snack
5 to 10 pretzels
2 celery stalks with 1 to 2 tablespoons salad dressing for dipping

Dinner
1 cup *Boiled Vegetables* over
1 to 2 cups *Linguine with Garlic and Oil*

Snack
1 apple
¾ cup of corn flakes
½ to 1 cup rice or almond milk

Nutrition Content For Day
Calories: 2,369
Fat: 84.5 g, 15.7 g saturated
Protein: 39.2 g
Potassium: 2,191 mg

Phosphorus: 338 mg

Recipes For The Day
Low Protein Shake
Ingredients:
1 cup blueberries
12 to 14 oz. of rice or almond milk
1 tbsp. of vanilla extract
You can add honey, essential amino acid powder, acacia fiber, oils especially fish and flaxseed.

Directions:
Blend ingredients until a smooth consistency. Adjust ingredient doses to desired amounts.

Boiled Vegetables
Directions:
1 to 2 cup of kidney-friendly vegetables. Boil vegetables till tender or as desired. Strain vegetables and season to taste. Drizzle 1 to 2 tbsps. of sesame oil over vegetables.

Linguine with Garlic and Oil
Ingredients:
1 lb. (16 oz.) of linguine
½ cup walnut oil
3 to 5 cloves garlic (sliced)
1 pinch dried chili pepper flakes
2 tbsp. dried parsley
1 tsp. fresh ground black pepper
1 tbsp. grated cheese

Directions:
Cook linguine following the package directions. Sauté sliced garlic cloves (add more garlic, to taste) in walnut oil over medium heat until golden brown. Remove garlic and set aside. Add dry pepper flakes, cook for an additional minute. Add parsley, cook 1 minute. Add cooked linguine, toss in garlic, arrange on serving platter, and sprinkle with black pepper and grated cheese.

Week 1, Day 7
Breakfast
1 to 2 cups oatmeal
You can add ½ to 1 cup of cranberries, blueberries, and other kidney friendly fruits

Lunch
Vegetarian Pita Sandwich
6 to 8 potato chips

Snack
¼ of an avocado with salad dressing
1 slice of bread with jam or butter

Dinner
1 to 2 cups *Thai-Style Pesto with Rice Pasta*

Snack
2 cups popcorn
4 strawberries

Nutrition Content For Day
Calories: 1,392
Fat: 60 g, 7.6 g saturated
Protein: 27 g
Potassium: 1,231 mg
Phosphorus: 193 mg, 27.5%
Sodium: 1,396 mg

Recipes For The Day
Pita Veggie Sandwich
Ingredients:
One regular pita bread
2 to 4 tbsp. of babaganoush (can be purchased at Mediterranean or Middle Eastern markets)
2 to 3 slices of cucumber
1 or 2 slices of tomato
2 or 3 lettuce leaves
2 slices of onion
1 tsp. of hot sauce

You can add ranch dressing or mustard sauce and desired seasonings

Directions:
You can either cut pita in half, or gently cut a small part of the top, creating a "pocket." Fill the pocket in this order with babaganoush, cucumber slices, onion, hot sauce, tomatoes, lettuce, sprinkle some seasonings. Top it with ranch, mustard sauce or both and some more hot sauce if desired.

Thai-Style Pesto with Rice Pasta
Ingredients:
1 lb. rice pasta, penne or wide noodles
1/3 cup fresh basil leaves
¼ cup dried basil leaves
2 tbsp. tamari
1 large cloves garlic, pasted
½ lime, juiced
½ Chile pepper, seeded
¼ cup extra-virgin olive oil
Toasted sesame oil, for drizzling

Directions:
Bring a large pot of water to a boil. Add the pasta and cook to al dente. Save water for later. Place the fresh and dried basil, tamari, garlic, lime juice, and chile into a food processor and "pulse" into a paste. Drizzle in the extra-virgin olive oil. Pour the pesto into a large bowl and add a splash of the saved pasta water. Drain the pasta, add to the sauce and toss to combine. Drizzle with sesame oil.

Week 2, Day 1
Breakfast
2 to 3 - 5 to 6 inch *Low Protein Pancakes*

Lunch
1 cup *German Red Cabbage* over 1 to 2 cups rice

Snack
1 cup *Low Protein Trail Mix*

Dinner

Pita Veggie Sandwich #2
1 pear

Snack
3 cups popcorn

Nutrition Content For Day
Calories: 1,392
Fat: 60 g, 7.6 g saturated
Protein: 27 g
Potassium: 1,231 mg
Phosphorus: 193 mg, 27.5%
Sodium: 1,396 mg

Recipes For The Day
Low Protein Pancakes
Directions:
Make pancakes with rice, tapioca or potato flour. Replace the egg with sesame oil, but start with a few tablespoons at a time until you meet the desired consistency. Use almond or rice milk in place of cow or goat milk. You also can add ½ to 1 cup kidney-friendly fruit, maple syrup, jam, butter, cinnamon to pancakes.

German Red Cabbage (Boiled)
Ingredients:
3 cup shredded red cabbage
2 medium unpeeled apples, cubed
¼ cup cider vinegar
1/8 tsp. pepper
1 dried bay leaf
1 tbsp. sesame oil
Dash of caraway seed

Directions:
Place butter, cabbage, apples, and sugar into a large pot. Pour in the vinegar, butter, water, bay leaf, pepper, and caraway seed.

Bring to a boil over medium-high heat, then reduce heat to low, cover, and simmer until the cabbage is tender, 1 to 1 ½ hours

Protein Trail Mix
Ingredients:
¼ cup dried cranberries
1/3 cup dried apple rings, diced
2 to 3 cup rice cracker/snacks, pretzels, etc.

Directions:
Mix all ingredients in large bowl and serve at room temperature.

Pita Veggie Sandwich #2
Ingredients:
1 pita bread
1 to 2 tbsp. mayo
2 tbsp. feta cheese
4 to 10 lettuce leaves
1 to 2 slices tomato
¼ cup alfalfa sprouts
1 small to medium roasted pepper
1 thin slice red onion

Directions:
You can cut the pita in half, or gently cut a small part of the top open section to create a "pocket." Fill the pocket in this order, spread mayo, feta cheese, onion, tomatoes, lettuce, and sprinkle some seasonings if desired.

Week 2, Day 2
<u>**Breakfast**</u>
1 to 1 ½ cups fruit salad
1 waffle with butter, maple syrup, jam, etc.
½ cup almond or rice milk.

<u>**Snack**</u>
4 ounces of yogurt
Dairy products are not to be consumed often

<u>**Lunch**</u>
1 to 2 cups *Pasta Vegetable Soup*
2 pieces of Italian bread (1" wide);
you can add oil-based dipping sauce

Snack
2 rice cakes with 1 to 2 tablespoons of jam

Dinner
5 to 6 inch of ¼ a loaf of *Garlic Bread*
8 *Boiled Asparagus Spears*

Snack
1 cup popcorn

Nutrition Content For Day
Calories: 1,876
Fat: 44.6, 15.7 g saturated
Protein: 34.2 g
Potassium: 1,077 mg
Phosphorus: 763 mg

Recipes For The Day
Pasta Vegetable Soup
Ingredients:
1 to 1 ½ cup of vegetable broth
3 to 4 ½ cup of water
1 cup carrots, sliced
¼ tsp. ground black pepper
1 cup celery, sliced
½ cup red pepper, chopped
½ cup radishes
1 clove garlic, minced
1 tsp. dried basil leaves
1 ½ cup uncooked spiral macaroni
½ cup onion, diced

Directions:
In large saucepan, over medium-high heat, bring water, vegetable broth, red pepper, garlic, carrots, celery, onion, basil, radishes and black pepper to a boil. Stir in macaroni, simmer 10 minutes. If needed, cook 5 more minutes or until pasta is done.

Garlic Bread
Ingredients:
1 16 oz. loaf of Italian bread or French bread
5 tbsp. unsalted butter, softened

1 large cloves of garlic, smashed and minced
1 heaping tbsp. of dried parsley
1 tbsp. oil (walnut, olive, canola, etc) of choice

Directions:
Cut bread into ½" slices. In a small bowl, mix butter, oil, garlic, and pepper. Spread the mixture evenly on the bread slices.

Place bread slices in a toaster oven and toast until butter is bubbling and edges of bread are brown. You can also make this bread in the oven. Reassemble the bread slices to form the loaf and wrap in heavy duty foil, leaving foil open at the top. Place in 450°F degree oven for 10-12 minutes until butter is melted and bread is crisp.

Boiled Asparagus Spears
Directions:
In large skillet, bring 1 inch of water to a boil, add asparagus in one layer. Cook until tender, about 5 minutes for medium and 7 minutes for jumbo. Drain, and transfer to a serving platter. Sprinkle with salt and pepper, and top with a pat of butter.

Week 2, Day 3
Breakfast
4 inch bagel with butter
Low Protein Shake

Lunch
1 to 1 ½ cups *Boiled White Turnips & Vegetables* over 1 to 2 cups rice, season to desired taste

Snack
1 apple
10 tortilla chips

Dinner
Veggie Burger
1 cup popcorn

Snack
1 cup *Fruit Salad*
4 to 5 melba toast

Nutrition Content For Day
Calories: 1,621
Fat: 44.7 g, 13.6 g saturated
Protein: 36.2 g
Potassium: 1,310 mg
Phosphorus: 219 mg

Recipes For The Day
Fruit Salad
Ingredients:
½ medium apple, diced in small pieces
½ cup blueberries
½ cup blackberries
8 grapes
¼ cup raspberries
2 to 3 tbsp. grape juice
You can add honey or vanilla extract, if desired

Directions:
In a large bowl, combine all ingredients. Gently toss to coat all fruits. Keep in refrigerator and serve chilled.

Boiled White Turnips & Vegetables
Ingredients:
4 or 5 white turnips
½ cup diced onion
½ cup celery, chopped
2 tbsp. canola oil
¾ cup water

Directions:
Cut raw turnips in pieces and boil in water until tender. Mix in celery and onion and canola oil in the water. Cook until done. Add butter, toss lightly and put over rice.

Veggie Burger
Ingredients:
1 veggie burger patty that is 3 to 5 grams of protein
1 hamburger bun
1 to 2 lettuce leaves

1 slice tomato
1 slice onion
Seasoning and condiments can
be added, such as mayo, etc.

Directions:
Place veggie patty on hamburger bun, top with lettuce, tomato, onion, and seasonings/condiments. Close with other hamburger bun.

Low Protein Shake
Ingredients:
¾ cup blueberries
1/3 banana
12 to 14 oz. of rice or almond milk
1 tbsp. of vanilla extract
You can add honey, essential amino acid powder, acacia fiber, oils especially fish and flaxseed.

Week 2, Day 4
Breakfast
Low Protein French Toast
You can add butter, maple syrup, etc.
12 cherries on the side or add fruit to French Toast
1 cup rice or almond milk

Snack
1 small roll toasted with 2 tablespoon jam

Lunch
Low Protein Coleslaw Sandwich
1 cup watermelon

Snack
1 peach
1 ounce potato chips, about 6 to 10 chips

Dinner
1 to 2 cups *Apple Macaroni Salad*

Snack
6 *Graham Cracker Desserts*

Nutrition Content For The Day
Calories: 1,463
Fat: 49.5 g, 11.5 g saturated
Protein: 31 g
Potassium: 1,618 mg
Phosphorus: 413 mg

Recipes For The Day
Low Protein French Toast
Ingredients:
1 cup rice or almond milk
2 tbsp. flour
1 tbsp. nutritional yeast flakes
1 tsp. vanilla extract
Pinch nutmeg
6 slices bread of choice

Directions:
Set aside break slices. Mix all the other ingredients in a shallow bowl. Dip the bread slices into the milk mixture and place on a nonstick griddle, until light brown on both sides. You can bake bread on a greased cookie sheet in a 400°F oven until light gold on both sides, turning once.

Low Protein Coleslaw Sandwich
Ingredients:
2 slices bread of choice
1 tbsp. mayonnaise
4 to 8 tbsp. of traditional coleslaw
1 soy cheese slice
1 tsp. of lemon

Directions:
Apply mayonnaise to each slice. Add coleslaw, slice of soy cheese and lemon. Cover with other slice of bread. Serve cold.
Note: Do not use soy cheese often in your diet. It can be included every so often for variety.

Apple Macaroni Salad
Ingredients:
½ cup pasta
1 cup diced unpeeled apples
2 tbsp. chopped celery
2 tbsp. dried cranberries
2 tbsp. kidney-friendly oil/vinegar dressing

Directions:
Cook, rinse, and drain pasta according to package directions. In a medium bowl, combine the cooked pasta with the rest of the ingredients and toss lightly.

Graham Cracker Desserts
Ingredients:
1 regular graham cracker
¼ tsp. butter
½ tsp. cinnamon

Directions:
Spread the graham cracker with butter. Sprinkle the cinnamon over the cracker. Bake for 10 minutes at 275°F degrees. Let cool.

Week 2, Day 5
Breakfast
1 to 2 *Low Protein Muffins* toasted with jam or butter
1 cup rice milk
½ orange

Snack
1 cup *Low Protein Trail Mix*

Lunch
1 to 2 cups *Israeli Couscous with Chard*

Snack
1 rice cake with jam

Dinner
½ cup boiled broccoli over
1 to 2 cups rice

8 to 10 *Low Protein Onion Rings*

Snack
1 *Honey Lemon Glazed Pear*

Nutrition Content For Day
Calories: 1,549
Fat: 37 g, 8.9 g saturated
Protein: 35.2 g
Potassium: 1,139 mg
Phosphorus: 333 mg

Recipes For The Day
Low Protein Muffins
Ingredients:
1 ½ cup all-purpose flour
¾ cup cornmeal
½ cup sugar
3 tbsp. baking powder
1 tsp. baking soda
orange zest from one orange
1 cup raspberries, fresh (or frozen)
1¼ cup almond milk
1 tbsp. apple cider vinegar
¼ cup oil
1 tsp. vanilla extract

Directions:
Preheat oven to 400°F degrees for 15 minutes. Grease or line a 12-cup muffin tin with paper liners. Mix together the almond milk and vinegar; set aside for a couple of minutes until it curdles. In a large bowl combine together the dry ingredients including the orange zest. In a separate bowl, take 2 tablespoons of this mixture and combine it with the berries. This will avoid the berries from sinking to the bottom of the muffins.

In another bowl whisk together the curdled milk mixture, oil and vanilla extract. Gently fold in the wet ingredients into the dry mixture. Stir in the berries. Do not over mix the batter. Spoon the batter into the prepared muffin tins, about two-thirds full. Sprinkle some sugar on top of the muffins. Bake for about 15-20 minutes or until a toothpick inserted in the center of the muffin comes out clean. Transfer to a wire rack and let it cool for at least 5 minutes before removing from the pan.

Israeli Couscous with Chard
Ingredients:
¾ cup chicken broth
1 cup water
1 ¼ cup Israeli couscous or regular couscous
walnut oil for drizzling
1 ½ large cloves garlic
1 tsp. whole white cumin
1 dried red chili pepper (optional)
2 cup chopped chard
¼ cup chicken broth
1 tbsp. balsamic vinegar

Directions:
Heat the broth to boiling in a small saucepan. Stir in the grains and lower the heat to a simmer. Cover and cook for about 10-14 minutes. Remove the lid and set aside.

Heat the olive oil in a large, heavy skillet over medium-low heat. Sliver the garlic and cook it on low heat with the cumin and chili pepper until soft and fragrant. Don't let it brown.

Add the chopped chard and turn the heat to medium. Sauté for about 5 minutes or until it begins to wilt. Add the cooked couscous and the ¼ cup of broth. Cook for another five minutes, stirring, until the broth has cooked off and the chard is fully wilted. Add seasonings, vinegar, and serve.

Low Protein Onion Rings
Ingredients:
2 Vidalia onions (about a pound), or other sweet onion like Walla Walla
½ cup plus 2 tbsp. all-purpose flour
2 tbsp. corn starch
1 cup cold almond milk
1 tsp. apple cider vinegar
1 cup bread crumbs
1 tsp. kosher salt

2 tsp. walnut oil

Directions:
Preheat oven to 450°F. Line a rimmed 12×18 baking sheet with parchment paper, spray with cooking spray and set aside.

Slice onions into ¾ inch thick rings. Separate the rings and place in a bowl.
Gather two bowls: one for batter and one for breading (large wide cereal bowls should work.)

In one bowl, pour in flour and cornstarch. Add about half of the almond milk and stir vigorously with a fork to dissolve. Add the rest of the almond milk and the apple cider vinegar, and stir. Set aside.

In the other bowl, mix together the bread crumbs and salt. Drizzle in the oil and use your fingertips to mix it up well.

From left to right, dip onion slice into the flour and gently shake excess.

Spoon breadcrumbs over the onion, coating completely. Carefully transfer each onion to a single layer on the baking sheet. Spray rings lightly with cooking spray and bake for 8 minutes. Flip, and bake another 6 minutes. Rings should be varying shades of brown and crispy. Taste one to check for doneness. Serve as soon as possible. With low salt ketchup if you like.

Honey Lemon Glazed Pear
Ingredients:
¼ cup melted butter
1/3 cup honey
4 medium ripe to firm pears
½ lemon (for zesting and juicing)

Directions:
Heat oven to 450°F degrees. Grate and juice lemon. You should have 3 to 4 tablespoons juice. In a small bowl, whisk together butter, honey, and the lemon juice.

Peel the pears if you like, but it is not necessary. Cut the pears in half lengthwise. Using a melon baller or a ½ teaspoon measuring spoon, neatly scoop out the core.

Place the pears in an 8 by 10 inch glass baking dish, pan or ceramic pan. Pour glaze mixture over the pears, allowing it to flow into the pan. In the cavity of each pear half, sprinkle some grated lemon zest.

Bake pears for 10 minutes, and baste with glaze. Bake for another 10 minutes, or until pears are very tender. Baste again with glaze and cool slightly. Serve warm.

Week 2, Day 6
Breakfast
1 serving of *Vegan Overnight Oats*
1 cup rice or almond milk

Snack
1 cup *Caramelized Rice Crispies*

Lunch
Low Protein Wrap

Snack
5 to 10 pretzels
6 to 8 *Dried Apple Rings*

Dinner
1 to 2 cups *Low Protein Fettuccine Alfonso*

Snack
4 to 5 pieces of *Rice Crispy Clusters*

Nutrition Content For Day
Calories: 1,648
Fat: 49.7 g, 14.1 g saturated
Protein: 34.3 g
Potassium: 1,101 mg
Phosphorus: 255 mg

Recipes For The Day
Vegan Overnight Oats
Ingredients:
½ cup regular oats
1 cup almond milk, and more if needed
1-2 tbsp. Metamucil™ fiber
½ cup blueberries
½ cup blackberries
¼ tsp. pure vanilla extract

Directions:
Mix together all ingredients in a bowl and place in fridge overnight. In the morning, add your desired toppings and serve.

Caramelized Rice Crispies
Ingredients:
¼ cup brown sugar
2 tbsp. water
2 cup rice crispies

Directions:
In a large skillet, bring the sugar and water to a boil over medium high heat. Boil for 1 minute, until sugar is dissolved completely. Sprinkle the rice crispies over the syrup, stirring gently to coat. Continue stirring gently over medium high heat until the cereal is a medium golden brown, about 4 ½ minutes.

Remove from heat and immediately transfer the caramelized cereal to a baking sheet to cool, spreading out into a single layer. When cool, break up the clumps and store at room temperature in an airtight container.

Low Protein Wrap
Ingredients:
1 to 2 tbsp. of matchstick cut carrots
1 to 2 tbsp. of chopped seeded tomato
1 to 2 tbsp. of chopped avocado
1 to 2 tbsp. sliced seeded cucumber
1 to 2 tbsp. grated radishes
1 to 2 tbsp. ranch dressing

1 (4 to 6 inch) flour or corn tortillas

Directions:
Combine first 6 ingredients in a large bowl. Add dressing to vegetable mixture; toss gently to coat.

Warm tortillas according to package directions. Spoon 3/4 cup vegetable mixture down center of each tortilla; roll up.

Low Protein Fettuccine Alfonso
Ingredients:
1 ½ cup corn kernels (fresh, frozen or canned)
1 ½ cup rice milk
2 tbsp. tahini
1 tbsp. onion granules
1 lb. fettuccine
cracked black pepper
additional seasonings if desired

Directions:
If using frozen corn, thaw and drain it well. Place corn, milk, tahini, and seasonings in blender and process until completely smooth. (This may take several minutes to completely pulverize the corn.)

Pour the blended mixture into a medium saucepan and heat on low to medium heat. While sauce is heating, boil fettuccine in large pasta pot until tender. Drain well and return to pot. Add 1 teaspoon of hot sauce if desired, and toss until noodles are evenly coated. Serve immediately, topping portions with a generous amount of cracked pepper.

Rice Crispy Clusters
Ingredients:
4 squares chocolate bar
1 ½ cup rice crispy cereal

Directions:
Prepare a baking sheet by lining it with waxed paper; set aside. Microwave chocolate in a microwave safe bowl on high power for 2 to 3 minutes, stirring once or twice.

Stir in cereal and mix well. Drop by teaspoon onto prepared baking sheet and let cool until firm. Can be stored in an air tight container for up to 3 weeks.

Week 2, Day 7
Breakfast
1 to 2 cups *Breakfast Rice Pudding*

Snack
Low Protein Shake #2

Lunch
Avocado Reuben

Snack
1 apple
½ to ¾ cup cereal

Dinner
1 cup boiled kidney-friendly vegetables over
1 to 2 cups of pasta with garlic and oil

Snack
1 cup *Strawberry Lemonade Granita*

Nutrition Content For Day
Calories: 1,827
Fat: 53 g, 18 g saturated
Protein: 38 g
Potassium: 1,298 mg
Phosphorus: 287 mg

Recipes For The Day
Breakfast Rice Pudding
Ingredients:
2 cup cooked rice
1 to 1 ½ cup vanilla rice milk
2 tbsp. raisins
2 tbsp. maple syrup
1 tsp. vanilla extract
¼ tsp. cinnamon

Directions:
In a medium-size saucepan, combine all ingredients and bring to a slow simmer. Cook uncovered, stirring occasionally for about 20 minutes, or until thick. Serve hot or cold.

Avocado Reuben
Ingredients:
2 slices rye bread
Mustard, as desired
Thousand Island dressing
1/3 small avocado, pitted, peeled, and mashed
¼ cup sauerkraut

Directions:
Spread one slice of bread with some mustard, the other slice with Thousand Island dressing.

Place the bread slices, dry side down, in a lightly walnut oiled skillet. Top one slice with avocado and the other with sauerkraut. Over medium heat, grill the sandwich until lightly browned and hot, about 5 minute. Sandwich together or leave open.

Lemonade Granita
Ingredients:
2 ¼ cup water
½ cup sugar
½ cup fresh lemon juice (from 1 ½ lemons)
½ cup puréed strawberries

Directions:
In a medium saucepan, bring water and sugar to a simmer over medium-high heat until sugar is dissolved. Remove from heat; add lemon juice and strawberry purée.

Pour mixture into a shallow pan or dish and put in the freezer. Stir every 30 minutes with a fork until all of the liquid is frozen. Remove from freezer 20 to 30 minutes before serving.

Essential Amino Acid Products

Supplement Companies and Products

The following pages list supplement companies and the essential amino acid products they offer. As well as how many pills or how much powder to use to meet your nutritional needs.

The amounts listed are assuming you will use that one product to meet your nutritional needs. You can mix and match companies. For example, in the morning you may want to take an essential amino acid powder and at lunch take the pills.

There are many places to purchase supplements, the sites listed below are some online resources.

Where To Purchase Essential Amino Acid Supplements

You can contact healthy kidney inc for any supplement purchases you require. The websites below often carry the mentioned products

http://www.vitacost.com/
http://www.amazon.com/
http://www.camformulas.com/
http://www.rockwellnutrition.com/
http://www.luckyvitamin.com/
http://www.iherb.com/

Companies and Products

Essential Amino Acids

Healthy Kidney Inc.
501 North Avenue, Ground Floor
Wood-Ridge, NJ 07075
1-800-927-1738
https://www.healthykidneyinc.com

Product: Pure Kidney Amino Acid Tablets. Take 5 tablets daily or as directed by physician.

NOW Foods
395 S. Glen Ellyn Road
Bloomingdale, IL 60108
1-888-669-3663
http://www.nowfoods.com/

Product: Amino-9 Essential Powder
1 ¾ to 2 teaspoons one to three times per day.

International Nutrition Research Center
7900 Los Pinos Circle
Coral Gables, FL 33143
305-666-9222
http://www.masteraminoacidpattern.com/inrc/index.php

Product: Master Amino Acid Pattern (MAP)
Take 7 pills per day.

Note: 500-1000mg of L-histidine, found in one pill, should be taken daily with Master Amino Acid Pattern.

Core4 Nutrition
70 SW Century Drive
Suite 100-230
Bend, OR 97702
1-888-371-1033
https://core4nutrition.com

Product: Fundaminos Powder
Take 7 grams per day. One and half scoops in 8 to 12 ounces of water per day.

Note: 500-1000mg of L-histidine, found in one pill, should be taken daily with Fundaminos.

Kion Aminos
3980 N Broadway
Suite 103-183
Boulder, CO 80304
855-387-KION (5466)
https://getkion.com

Product: Kion Aminos Essential Amino Acids Powder
Take one and a half scoops in 8 to 12 ounces of water.
Note: 500-1000mg of L-histidine, found in one pill, should be taken daily with Kion.

Keto Analogues of Essential Amino Acid Companies

Contact each company about their products

Ketorena
1-844-980-9933
sales@nephcentric.com
http://www.ketorena.com

Kidneyhood.org/Albutrix
8383 Greenway Blvd.
Middleton, WI 53562
Tel: 800-441-1045
Email:info@kidneyhood.org

Low Protein Food Companies

Going very low protein can be difficult for some. The companies below provide premade food that is very low in protein.

When choosing low protein products from the companies listed, it's best to consume products with zero or minimal amounts of hydrogenated oils and sugar. If you find yourself very limited in choices remember it is best to eat low protein as opposed to eliminating hydrogenated oils and sugar.

If you are a diabetic choose the lowest sugar products available. This is a partial list of very low protein food companies available. You can search the internet to find other companies and products. List provided by http://www.pkupag.org

http://www.cambrookefoods.com/
They have their own brand of pastas, breads, snacks, baking mixes, prepared foods, mock high-protein foods, recipes, books and reference.

http://www.dietspecupcom/
They have their own brand of baking mixes, breads, desserts & snacks, pasta, mock high-protein foods, quick mix entrees and frozen items.

http://www.ener-g.com/
They have their own brand of baking mixes, breads including some unique styles, desserts & snacks, pasta, mock high-protein foods, soup broths, egg replacer, wheat starch, almond and chocolate bark.

http://www.med-diet.com/
Unimix baking mix, breads, desserts & snacks, pasta, most items listed as large quantity purchase only.

http://www.medicalfood.com/
This is Applied Nutrition. They offer Maddy's brand cereals and snacks, as well as Energy Option energy bars.

http://www.myspecialdiet.com/
SHS, Loprofin, and Wel-Plan products including baking mixes, breads, cereal, desserts & snacks, pasta, recipes, books and software, diet management tools, information, articles and message board.

http://www.tasteconnections.com/
They have their own brand of baking mixes and supply recipes and cooking tips.

Vegetarian Diet for Kidney Disease Introduction

The Vegetarian Diet for Kidney Disease

A vegetarian, plant based, diet has shown to slow down or stop renal disease from progressing. It can also prevent problems that often arise in renal disease such as high blood pressure, high cholesterol, inflammation, digestive issues, etc.

In a vegetarian diet the amino acids that make up plant based proteins, as opposed to animal proteins, create less stress on the kidneys, improving kidney health. Vegetarian foods create less pressure on the kidney and allow better glucose control, improving diabetes, and decreasing proteinuria.

Most vegetarians fall into one of the following categories:

- Lacto-vegetarians - This group excludes eggs, but consumes milk and other dairy products in addition to plant foods.

- Lacto-ovo vegetarians - This group consumes eggs, milk, dairy products and plant foods.

- Pesco-vegetarians - This group eats fish for health reasons, in addition to eating plant foods, dairy products and eggs.

- Vegan - This group consumes only plant foods and no animal products.

This Vegetarian Diet for Renal Disease falls under the category of a vegan diet with the exception of small amounts of mayo.

This is a 2-week vegetarian diet plan, including recipes and tips for eating out. You can mix and match the meal plan days to your liking and don't have to consume as many snacks as listed or as much food.

Making your own meals and snacks

There are many more menu and snack options available aside from what is included in this book. When making your own dishes you can modify other recipes by taking out protein foods such as dairy, eggs, meats, etc., and replacing with rice or almond milk, acceptable nuts, beans, seeds, soy products, oils, and small amounts of starches and flour. Also, many vegan recipes only need to be slightly modified or can be used as is.

Overview & Benefits of the Diet

Dietary management of renal disease is the core to improving your kidney health. Diet is the most important factor in preserving and improving the kidneys. Without a therapeutic diet, most efforts to preserve and improve your kidneys will have little long term effect.

A vegetarian diet for renal disease has been used for many decades. However, in recent years with new research conducted, I have modified this traditional diet with more healing and therapeutic foods and options.

This vegetarian diet comprises plant based protein along with low to moderate phosphorus intake, low to moderate potassium, low sodium, higher alkaline, and is a high fiber diet.

Dietary Protein

Dietary protein intake results in a faster rate of declining kidney function. This is because protein results in the accumulation of nitrogen waste products, urea, hydrogen ions, phosphates, and inorganic ions which have to be eliminated or regulated by the kidney. Dietary protein lost during renal disease (proteinuria) has also been shown to create inflammation further damaging the kidney.

Healthy kidneys can handle normal to large amounts of dietary protein, and keep the body in balance. When kidney disease is present, filtering out these waste products puts an increased stress on the kidneys. This leads to eventual loss of function.

Consuming a vegetarian diet with vegetarian protein sources takes the stress of performing these functions off of the kidneys leading to improving, slowing or arresting the kidney disease. It also improves symptoms of kidney disease including uremia, because fewer toxins are produced from vegetarian sources of protein.

The most important part of this diet is to keep your protein consumption from vegetarian sources between 0.6 grams to 0.8 grams of protein per kilogram of body weight per day (0.6g to 0.8g of protein x kilogram (kg) b.w./day). Keeping your daily protein consumption within this amount has shown to have benefits for type 1 and type 2 diabetes and other forms of kidney disease.

Low Phosphorus

Phosphorus is another important mineral that the kidneys need to keep regulated. In kidney disease, phosphorus levels can become elevated leading to complications with the skeletal system (bones), the body's energy production, and cell functioning. High levels also put more stress on the kidneys, forcing them to work harder which leads to a faster decline in function. Luckily, most absorbable phosphorus is contained in protein foods. Phosphorus in vegetarian foods is only 50% absorbed.

Low to Moderate Potassium

Potassium is one of the main minerals of the body. It plays a critical role in heart functioning through muscular contraction. The kidneys are responsible for excreting 90% of the potassium from the body. In renal disease, there may be either too little potassium or too much (too much is known as hyperkalemia). It's much more common to have hyperkalemia in kidney disease.

Hyperkalemia can lead to dysrhythmias (irregular heartbeats) and cardiac arrest. This along with high potassium levels may cause further damage to the kidneys. This is why a low to moderate potassium diet is being suggested.

Low Sodium

Sodium is essential for many body functions including regulating the blood pressure and blood volume, helping transmit impulses for nerve function, muscle contractions, and regulating the acid-alkaline (*aka.* acid-base) balance of blood and body fluids.

When kidney disease is present, extra sodium can build up in the body leading to fluid accumulation. This can cause swollen ankles, puffiness, a rise in blood pressure, shortness of breath, and/or fluid around your heart and lungs which can lead to heart failure. Keeping sodium levels low is important to maintaining overall health with kidney disease. Salt should never be added to foods. Keep sodium levels to 1500-2000mg per day.

Higher Alkaline

The kidneys maintain the acid-alkaline balance of the body (Ph level). When too much acid builds up in the body from acidic foods and the kidneys cannot keep the balance, the results are inflammation, chronic illness and worsening of kidney function.

This is why a higher alkaline diet is preferred. Every food is either considered alkaline or acidic, so maintaining a higher amount of alkaline foods will help take the stress off your kidneys.

High Fiber

A high fiber diet of 25 to 35 grams per day from food and supplements has shown to slow and improve kidney disease. Fiber has anti-inflammatory benefits and clears toxins out of the gastrointestinal tract which build up in renal disease. In order to achieve a high fiber diet without the additional potassium from fruits and vegetables, a supplement may be introduced.

Vegetarian

Why vegetarian? All animal sources of food (dairy, eggs, fish, chicken, meats including beef, lamb, goat, etc.) have shown to decrease kidney function once there is damage. The reason is that after digestion of animal proteins, more urea and toxins need to be filtered by your kidneys.

Vegetarian sources produce fewer toxins and have shown to delay loss of kidney function and in many cases improve it. Also, nutrients like phosphorus aren't readily absorbed from vegetarian sources of food.

Anti-Inflammatory & Anti-Oxidant

This diet will have many healthy, good anti-inflammatory fats and other foods which have been shown to help kidney disease. For example, sesame oil has been shown to help protect and help injured kidneys recover because of the anti-inflammatory and anti-oxidant benefits. This is why anti-inflammatory and anti-oxidant foods are important.

Vegetarian Diet Kidney Friendly Food List

The below foods are considered very kidney friendly. They are low in potassium, phosphorus, and some have therapeutic value such as anti-inflammatory and anti-oxidant benefits to combat kidney damage.

Frozen, Fresh and Canned Foods
It is best to use fresh or frozen foods because of the lower salt content of fresh foods and, in most cases, lower potassium content of frozen foods compared to canned foods. But the higher sodium content of frozen and canned foods, and the added sugar, often makes them undesirable. If you can, find frozen and canned foods without salt and added sugar.

Fats and Oils
Any oils can be used, but the below have shown benefits for kidney disease

Sesame seed oil and flax seed oil
These two oils have shown the most benefit, aside from fish oil, when kidney disease is present. You should avoid cooking with flax seed oil, as it can become a source of free radicals when heated.

Canola oil, coconut oil and walnut oil
These three oils have shown some benefit in kidney disease.

Extra virgin olive oil
This oil has shown healthy benefits to your cardiac and vascular system. There is no research showing harm or benefit to kidney disease, so it can be added in your diet.

Butter
Butter has not been shown to be either harmful or beneficial to the kidneys. Consider it neutral and so small amounts are

acceptable. However, butter and mayo should be your last choice for fats and should be avoided if there is high cholesterol.

Vinegars, Salt, Seasonings and Condiments

Vinegars
All vinegars are acceptable with kidney disease; make sure no salt is added.

Salt, Seasonings and Condiments
Avoid table salt and any seasonings that have the word "salt or sodium," and avoid salt substitutes (they contain potassium) and any seasonings with potassium. Purchase the lowest sodium foods you can and don't add salt to any foods. Most other seasonings are acceptable.

List of Seasonings and Condiments
Allspice, basil, bay leaf, caraway seed, chives, cilantro, cinnamon, cloves, cumin, curry, dill, extracts (almond, lemon, lime, maple, orange, peppermint, vanilla, walnut), fennel, garlic powder, ginger, horseradish (root), lemon juice, low sodium hot sauce like Tabasco®, mustard, Mrs. Dash®, nutmeg, onion powder or flakes, oregano, paprika, parsley flakes, pepper (ground), pimentos, poppy seed, rosemary, saffron, sage, savory, sesame seeds, tarragon, thyme, turmeric, vegan mayo.

Salad Dressings
It is best to make your own with oil, vinegar, spices, and vegan mayo, for example. Some Russian, French, and Ranch dressings have low potassium and protein levels.

Jelly, Jams and Honey

Jelly, Jams and Honey
These are simple sugars that contain only small amounts of potassium, sodium or phosphorus when used in the amounts listed to consume.

You can have between two to five tablespoons per day. It is best to stay close to two tablespoons, and look for the least amount of sugar when purchasing jams and jellies.

Beverages

Water, Green Tea and Hibiscus Tea
Consume more of your beverages from water, green tea and hibiscus tea. You can consume 2 cups (16-24 ounces) of tea per day. Consuming green and hibiscus tea has shown to benefit the kidneys.

Chamomile and Black Tea
If you find you do not like green tea, you can substitute with 16-24 ounces per day of chamomile and black tea. They have some benefit for kidney disease, but not as much as green tea. Chamomile should be your first choice and black tea the second.

A Word about Teas
In the early stages of kidney disease (1, 2, and most likely all of stage 3) you can consume higher amounts of teas, but make sure you have your potassium checked before and after doing this.

Rice and Almond Milk
Rice milk and almond milk can be consumed because they are low in potassium, phosphorus and protein. It can be used as a replacement for milk in cooking or baking. Flavored varieties are available which have a little more potassium and phosphorus than non-flavored.

Fruits

Apple	Apple Sauce	Apple Butter
Apples, Dried	Blackberries	Blueberries
Cherries	Cranberries	Dried Cranberries
Grapes	Lemon	Lime
Pineapple	Plums	Raspberries
Strawberries	Tangerines	

Vegetables

Alfalfa Seeds, Sprouted Raw	Asparagus	Bean Sprouts
Cabbage	Corn	Cauliflower
Green Beans	Eggplant	Jicama
Leeks	Lettuce, all kinds	Mushrooms, shiitake
Onions	Peas, Green	Peppers, chili
Scallions	Radicchio	Radishes
Water Chestnuts	White Turnips	

Soy

When the option is available, soy products should be purchased as non-GMO. GMO stands for Genetically Modified Organisms. GMO soy products have shown to possibly create kidney damage. If GMO is out of your budget you can still consume soy products. The soy research showing positive benefits did not use non-GMO.

Soy milk – 8 ounce per day	Tofu	Tempeh
Edamame Beans		

Nuts & Seeds

Almond	Macadamia	Pecan
Walnut	Peanut Butter	Almond Butter
Chia Seeds	Pumpkin Seeds	Sesame Seeds
Flaxseeds – They are high in potassium but included because they have shown to be beneficial in kidney disease.		

Beans & Legumes

Black Beans	Black Eyed Peas	Fava Beans
Hummus	Babaghanoush	Mung Beans
Pinto Beans	Garbanzo/Chick Peas	

Breads/Cereals/Grains
Find the Lowest Salt, Sugar and Lowest Protein Products Made Up of the Grains Below

Whole Grains – Whole grains have higher amounts of phosphorus and potassium and should be avoided or limited in kidney disease. Choose refined grains which are usually listed on the package label as refined, enriched or have the word whole before the name of the grain.

However, in stages 1, 2, and 3 of kidney disease you can have more whole grains in your diet, provided your phosphorus and potassium levels are in mid-range.

Make Sure to Choose the Lowest Protein, Lowest Sugar and Unsalted or the lowest sodium products you can find for all foods listed. Remember to read all labels and check all products because every gram of protein, salt, and sugar will count.

Bread, Cereals and Grain Products

Wheat Flour	Bagels	Bread Sticks
Bulgur Wheat	Couscous	Crackers, Wheat
Croissants	Dinner Rolls or Hard Rolls	English Muffins
French Bread	Italian Bread	Light Rye
Melba Toast	Noodles	Oyster Crackers
Pancakes	Pasta, all kinds	Pita bread
Pretzels	Soft Wheat	Tortillas
Waffles	White/Wheat Bread	

Corn

Corn Flour/Meal	Corn Chips (unsalted)	Corn Grits
Corn Muffins	Corn Tortillas	Corn Pancakes, made with no eggs
Popcorn (unsalted)		

Rice

Rice Flour	Most White Rices	Rice Pasta
Rice Bread	Rice Cakes	Rice Crackers
Cassava, aka Tapioca or Yuca	Tapioca Flour/Starch, not the root vegetable	

Cassava, aka Tapioca or Yuca and Potatoes

Tapioca Flour/Starch, not the root vegetable
Potato Flour/Starch

Gluten Free Products

Some gluten free products are acceptable depending on the flour source used. Check protein content, sodium and, if labeled, potassium.

Breads	Pancakes
Waffles	Crackers

Cereals, Dry

Corn Flakes	Puffed Wheat	Rice Cereal
Other cereals with crisp, chex or puff in the name		

Cereals, Hot

Cream of Rice	Cream of Wheat	Grits
Malt-O-Meal	Wheat Farina	For more flavor, consider cinnamon, kidney friendly fruit or Tabasco® (a favorite for grits).

Soup Broths

Use a base of water or low potassium, low protein, low salt commercial brands and avoid drinking the broth.

Moderately Kidney-Friendly Foods and Beverages

These foods will have higher amounts of potassium and phosphorus, and if your levels of these two minerals are low or in the middle range on your lab work you can consume some of the additional foods below.

Beverages and Sweeteners

Juices

8 ounces (1 cup) of juices or below have acceptable amounts of potassium (100-150mg). Be mindful to not have too much juice in your diet as the potassium content can rise quickly. No more than 4 to 8 ounces per day.	Cranberry juice	Grape Juice bottled - 6 ounces maximum
Grape Juice Frozen	Crangrape Juice	Cranapple Juice
Lemonade	Pear Nectar	

Sweeteners

Maple Syrup

Natural Sweeteners

Stevia, aka Stevia Rebaudiana (Truvia™, PureVia™) is a zero calorie natural sweetener taken from herbaceous perennial plant from the genus Stevia Cav. Rebaudioside A and stevioside are steviol glycosides which are extracts taken from the leaves that have been used as natural sweeteners for over 20 years in South America, Brazil, and Japan. It has a Generally Recognized as Safe (GRAS) status as a general-purpose sweetener for food and drink by the FDA.

Research is promising as it has shown beneficial when renal disease and hypertension are present. Moderate amounts can be consumed, even in baking.

Condiments

Mayonnaise, 1-2 tbsp. per day

Fruits

Elderberries	Olives, find lowest sodium and if needed blanch (see below) or soak in water, a few hours to overnight, to reduce sodium content. Avoid if you need to restrict sodium.	Orange
Peaches	Pears	Honeydew
Watermelon		

Vegetables

Beets	Broccoli	Brussels Sprouts
Carrots	Celery	Collards
Mushrooms	Okra	Potato Chips
Squash	Sweet Potato, 1 small to medium, double boiled without skin if you need to keep potassium low	

Whole Grains

Whole grains contain many nutrients and can be considered kidney friendly, if your phosphorus and potassium levels are under control. If your phosphorus and potassium levels are out of range you should not consume whole grains and consume the grains in the kidney friendly list.

Amaranth	Brown Rice	Bulgur
Kamut	Millet	Oats
Whole Wheat	Rye	Sorghum
Spelt	Wild Rice	

Nuts & Seeds

Brazil Nut	Pine Nut	Sunflower

Beans & Legumes

Kidney Beans	Lentils

Unfriendly Kidney Foods List

Beverages

Fruit Juices, Soft Drinks, Coffee
Other fruit juices, not listed in kidney friendly foods and sodas/soft drinks should be avoided due to fructose (fruit sugar) intake, higher potassium and phosphorus levels. Fructose and sugar (mentioned below) added to soft drinks such as soda, ginger ale, etc., and other fruit juices have shown to create inflammation, contribute to high blood pressure, obesity, diabetes, and increase the risk of further damage to the kidneys.

Coffee
Coffee should be limited to 1, 8 ounce cup per day. Even though recent reports state that coffee can be beneficial in many diseases, further studies need to be conducted in CKD, and until then it should be limited. Coffee should be avoided in polycystic kidney disease.

Alcohol
Alcohol consumption should be avoided in CKD. If you want to have alcohol red wine is preferred for kidney disease.

Sweeteners and Artificial Sweeteners

Sugar/Sucrose
Sugar, *aka* sucrose should be minimized or eliminated in kidney disease. Sugar is very difficult to avoid as it's added to many products including breads. Small amounts are acceptable within the diet, but large amounts should be avoided by eliminating sugary beverages and large amounts of baked goods, cookies, cakes, pies, candies, etc.

High sugar/sucrose intake has shown to increase the risk of diabetes, worsen its condition, suppress the immune system, increase uric acid, decrease HDL (good) cholesterol, and increase symptoms attributed to Irritable Bowel Syndrome such as gas, bloating, and diarrhea.

Fructose and High-Fructose Corn Syrup
Fructose, a popular ingredient in beverages, and HFCS should be minimized or avoided, as the problems associated with sucrose and fructose apply to high fructose corn syrup as well.

Sugar Alcohols
Sugar alcohols such as sorbitol, erythritol, xylitol, mannitol, lactitol and maltitol. Not much is known about these sweeteners and their connection to kidney disease. Small amounts in combination with Stevia™ can be consumed, but they should be limited until further research is conducted.

Artificial Sweeteners
Avoid all artificial sweeteners as some have shown to be harmful to the nervous system and brain. They can raise the risk of cancer, and there is concern over their involvement in other health problems. Many artificial sweeteners have not been studied in relation to kidney disease and should be avoided until further research is conducted.

Here is a list of artificial sweeteners: Saccharin (Sweet'N Low®), SugarTwin®), Aspartame (NutraSweet®, Equal®), Acesulfame K (ACK, Sunett®, Sweet One®), Sucralose (Splenda®), and the recent Neotame.

Fruits and Vegetables

Avoid the exotic star fruit, as it has shown to be very toxic to the kidney. Other fruits, vegetables, as well as friendly and moderately-friendly kidney foods may be consumed in liberal quantities if your blood tests show your potassium levels are in range. The issue with these foods is the potassium content. If you need strict control over your potassium levels, then the fruits and vegetables not listed should be avoided.

Vegetarian Diet Plate Method
Use this as a guide for choosing portion size & balancing nutrients

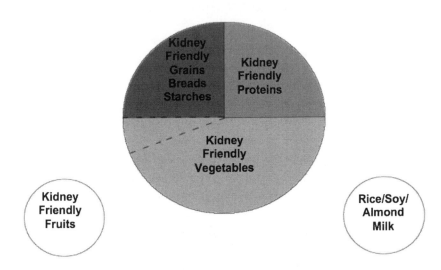

Additional Beverages: Water and Kidney Friendly Tea and Juices.

Dashed Lines: The space between the dashed lines can be varied according to your glucose numbers. If you have good blood sugar control and no elevated potassium levels, you can include more kidney friendly grains, breads and starches in that section. However, it is preferred to have kidney friendly vegetables between the dashed lines.

Vegetarian Diet Sample Menu Plan

This sample meal plan is based on a 175 pound person consuming 0.6, 0.7 or 0.8 grams of protein per kilogram of body weight per day which is 47, 55, and 63 grams of protein per day.

You will have to calculate your protein requirements and adjust the protein content per meal using the calculation on pages 22 through 24. You don't have to consume as many meals and snacks as listed. You can combine snacks with meals or eat less food than what is listed.

Week 1, Day 1
Breakfast
1 cup fresh sweet cherries
1 cup cooked oatmeal with 1 tablespoon peanut butter

Lunch
2 cups Black Bean Soup
¾ cup fresh pineapple

Snack
1 cup raw carrots
¼ cup hummus

Dinner
2 cups Pasta with Braised Broccoli and Tomato
1 cup steamed green beans
1 cup rice milk

Snack
1 ounce roasted unsalted almonds

Nutritional Content For The Day
Calories: 1694
Fat: 50.6 g, 6.1 g saturated
Carbohydrates: 266 g
Protein: 57.7 g
Potassium: 2,759 mg
Phosphorus: 508.2 mg

Recipes For The Day
Black Bean Soup
Ingredients:
6 cups vegetable broth
2 bell peppers, diced
2 small onions, diced
3 carrots, diced
2 ribs celery, diced
3 (15 oz) cans low-sodium black beans
½ teaspoon cumin
½ teaspoon chili powder

Directions:
In a large pot add the veggie broth, peppers, onions, carrots, and celery. Bring to a boil, reduce to a simmer and cook about 15 minutes, or until the carrots are tender. Add the black beans, cumin and chipotle powder. Taste for seasoning, add salt and pepper to taste. Bring back to a simmer (warm up the beans)

Pasta with Braised Broccoli and Tomatoes
Ingredients:
4 tablespoons extra virgin olive oil
1 head broccoli, cut into 1/2- to 1-inch florets, tough stems discarded
8 cloves garlic, thinly sliced
1 teaspoon dried oregano
1/2 teaspoon red chili flakes
1/2 cup dry white wine
2 (28-ounce) cans whole peeled tomatoes, roughly chopped, juice reserved
1 pound hearty short pasta, such as ziti or penne rigate
1/4 cup chopped fresh parsley leaves

Directions:
Heat olive oil in a large saucepan over medium heat until shimmering. Add broccoli and cook, stirring occasionally, until lightly browned in spots, about 5 minutes. Add garlic, oregano, and chili flakes. Cook, stirring constantly, until fragrant, about 30 seconds. Add wine and cook until slightly reduced, about 2 minutes. Add tomatoes. Bring to a boil, reduce to a simmer,

cover, and cook, stirring occasionally, until broccoli is completely tender and broken down, about 1 hour. Season to taste with salt.

Bring a large pot of salted water to a boil and cook pasta according to package directions. Drain and add to sauce. Add parsley leaves and stir to combine. Serve immediately, garnishing with additional extra virgin olive oil and parsley leaves as desired.

Week 1, Day 2
Breakfast
6 oz container of soy yogurt
1 cup blueberries
1 tablespoon chopped walnuts

Lunch
1 Vegan Veggie Pita
2 cups lettuce and cucumber salad
tablespoons dressing (1 tablespoon sesame oil, 1 tablespoon vinegar)

Snack
2 cups air popped popcorn
1 oz walnuts

Dinner
½ Southwestern Stuffed Spaghetti Squash

Snack
1 cup celery sticks
2 tbsp. almond butter

Nutritional Content For The Day
Calories: 1619
Fat: 75.9 g, 7.4 g saturated
Carbohydrates: 198 g
Protein: 51.7 g
Potassium: 2638 mg
Phosphorus: 584.5 mg

Recipes For The Day
Vegan Veggie Pita
Ingredients:
1 low-carb pita
1/3 cup chopped lettuce
¼ cup hummus
1/3 cup shredded carrots
1/3 cup shredded cucumber
Directions: Combine all ingredients in pita and serve

Southwest Style Stuffed Spaghetti Squash
Ingredients:
1 medium sized spaghetti squash
1 can low-sodium black beans
1 can whole kernel sweet corn, drained
1 large red or green bell pepper, diced
1 small yellow onion, diced
1/2 cup green onion, chopped
1 large handful fresh cilantro
1 jalapeño, diced

Directions:
Preheat oven to 400 F. Poke several holes in the skin of the squash to allow steam to escape while cooking. Place whole squash on a roasting pan and roast for 60 minutes.
Brown onion 4-5 minutes. Combine the beans, corn, red bell pepper, jalepeno, and cilantro.
Cut the squash in half, lengthwise. Using a large fork scrape out the flesh of the squash to make 'spaghetti' making sure to leave at least 1/2" on bottom and sides to create a "boat". Toss the spaghetti squash flesh in with the vegetable and bean mixture to combine. Scoop mixture into the spaghetti 'boats'. Place back in oven and roast for 10-15 minutes.
Garnish with cilantro and green onion.

Week 1, Day 3
Breakfast

Tropical Vegan Smoothie

Lunch
2 cups Rice and Chickpea Salad
1 cup bell pepper slices

Snack
½ cup trail mix (1/8 cup sunflower seeds, 1/8 cup dried cranberries, 1/8 cup
rice puffs, 1/8 cup raisins)

Dinner
1 Soy Protein Burger on low- carb bun
1 slice tomato, 1 slice lettuce, 1 slice onion
2 teaspoons mustard
1 small roasted sweet potato in 1 tablespoon olive oil

Snack
1 medium granny smith apple
1 tablespoon sunflower seed butter

Nutrition Content For The Day
Calories: 1,696
Fat: 51.3 g, 4.7 g saturated
Carbohydrates: 279 g
Protein: 46 g
Potassium: 1,977 mg
Phosphorus: 453.6 mg

Recipes For The Day
Tropical Vegan Smoothie
Ingredients:
12 oz rice milk
½ cup fresh pineapple
½ cup strawberries
½ cup ice

Directions: Blend all ingredients together and serve

immediately.

Rice and Chickpea Salad
Serves: 2
Ingredients:
1 cup uncooked rice (any color), rinsed and drained
2 cups water
1/4 cup walnut oil
2 teaspoons apple cider vinegar
Freshly ground black pepper
1 can low-sodium chickpeas
2 cups asparagus, steamed
1/2 small red onion, thinly sliced

Directions:
Place rice and water in a small saucepan. Bring to a boil, cover, and simmer over low heat. Simmer for about 15 minutes, or until all liquid is absorbed. Remove from heat and let stand for 5 minutes. Fluff rice with a fork and spread on a parchment-lined baking sheet to cool.

Whisk together walnut oil, vinegar and pepper.

Place rice, chickpeas, onion, and asparagus in a large bowl and stir gently to combine. Pour dressing over salad and toss gently to coat.

Soy Protein Burgers
Serves: 4
Ingredients:
3/4 cup boiling water
3/4 cup textured soy protein granules
1/4 cup oats
1/2 tsp onion powder
1/2 tsp garlic powder
3 tbsp. flour
1 tbsp. soy sauce
1 tbsp. ketchup
1/2 tsp. pepper

Directions:
Mix boiling water into textured soy protein granules and let sit for 15 minutes. In another bowl, mix together oats, onion powder, garlic powder, flour, soy sauce, ketchup, and pepper.
Once textured, soy protein is rehydrated, add oat mixture to textured soy protein and mix well. Cover and place in the fridge for 15 minutes to allow textured soy protein to firm up.
Remove textured soy protein and divide into quarters. With your hands, roll each quarter into a ball and flatten into a patty shape. Lightly brush each side with oil and add some oil to a large skillet. Heat oil until a drop of water sizzles, then add patties to the skillet. Cook 3-4 minutes on each side. Assemble the sandwich with lettuce, pickles, and tomatoes. Enjoy!

Week 1, Day 4
Breakfast

2 cups scrambled tofu and vegetables

Lunch
2 cups Easy Green Minestrone
1 cup blueberries

Snack
2 small tangerines
2 cups air popped popcorn

Dinner
Vegan Eggplant Sandwich
1 cup roasted green beans in 1 tablespoon olive oil

Snack
1 oz roasted pistachios

Nutrition Content For The Day
Calories: 2047
Fat: 63.4 g, 9.5 g saturated
Protein: 63 g
Potassium: 2728 mg
Phosphorus: 623 mg

Scrambled Tofu and Vegetables
Serves 2
Ingredients:
1 package of firm tofu
1 tablespoon olive oil
1 small chopped onion
1 cup sliced mushrooms
1 diced green pepper
½ tsp black pepper
½ tsp garlic powder

Directions: Heat oil over medium heat. Crumble tofu into small pieces in pan. Sauté tofu with all vegetables until soft.

Easy Green Minestrone
Serves: 4 (Makes 8 cups)
Ingredients:
2 tbsp. olive oil
1 yellow onion, diced
3 celery stalks, diced
2-3 cloves garlic, minced
1 tsp. fresh thyme (1/2 teaspoon dry)
1 bay leaf
6 cups vegetable or chicken broth
1 pound waxy red potatoes (4-5 small potatoes), cut into bite-sized pieces
1/2 pound green beans chopped
1 pound small-shaped pasta, like shells or elbow macaroni
6 oz. greens, like spinach, kale, or chard, chopped
1 (15-ounce) can white beans, like Great Northern
1 tsp black pepper

Directions:
In a large soup pot, warm the olive oil over medium heat. Add the onion, celery, and 1/4 teaspoon of salt, and cook until the onion and celery are soft and translucent, 8 to 10 minutes. Stir in the garlic, thyme, and bay leaf, and cook until the garlic is fragrant, about 30 seconds.

Add the chicken broth, the potatoes, and 1 teaspoon of salt to the pan. Increase the heat to high and bring the soup to a boil. Lower heat to medium-low and simmer the soup for 5 minutes.

Add the green beans and simmer for another 5 to 10 minutes, until both the potatoes and the green beans are tender.

While the soup is simmering, bring a pot of salted water to a boil and cook the pasta to al dente. Drain and set aside.
When the vegetables are tender, stir the greens and the white beans into the soup. Simmer until the greens are wilted and tender, 1 to 3 minutes. Taste and add additional salt and pepper if needed. To serve, add a scoop of pasta to each bowl and ladle the soup over top.

Vegan Eggplant Sandwich
Ingredients:
1 cup eggplant slices
1 tbsp. olive oil
6 inch French bread
1/3 cup tomato sauce
½ cup lentils
Directions: Stir-fry eggplant in olive oil until well cooked. Mix in lentils and tomato sauce. Serve over toasted French bread.

Week 1, Day 5
Breakfast
1 cup cherries
6 oz. vegan yogurt
1 tbsp. sunflower seeds

Lunch
2 cups kale, farro and chickpea salad
3 pieces melba toast

Snack
2 small plums

Dinner
2 cups Seared Tofu with Gingered Vegetables
1 cup cooked brown rice

Snack
1 small banana
2 tbsp. almond butter

Nutrition Content For The Day
Calories: 1879
Fat: 62 g, g saturated
Carbohydrates: 269 g
Protein: 43 g
Potassium: 2319 mg
Phosphorus: 469 mg

Chopped Kale, Farro & Chickpea Salad
Ingredients:
1/2 cup farro
1 bunch (about 10 ounces) Tuscan, Dino, or Lacinato kale
1 tbs. extra-virgin olive oil
1 tsp. red miso paste
2 tsp. lemon juice (about 1/2 lemon)
1 15.5-ounce can chickpeas, drained and rinsed

Directions:
Bring 2 cups of water to a boil in a 2-quart saucepan over medium-high heat. Add 1 teaspoon of salt and the farro, and stir.

Turn the heat to low and simmer uncovered for 25-30 minutes, until the farro is chewy and tender. Drain the farro from the excess liquid and set aside.

Wash and dry the kale leaves. Stack several leaves on top of each other and slice off the few inches of tough, fibrous stem from the bottoms. If desired, slice out the ribs (though I like the crunch these ribs add to the salad). Roughly chop the kale leaves into bite-sized pieces. Repeat stacking and slicing the remaining leaves of kale.

Transfer the chopped kale to a big mixing bowl. Whisk together the olive oil, miso paste, and lemon juice. Pour over the kale leaves. Use your hands to work the dressing into the kale leaves. Continue massaging the leaves until the kale has softened and feels silky, 1-2 minutes. Pour the farro and the drained chickpeas over the kale and toss to combine. Taste and add a sprinkle of salt or another squeeze of lemon if desired.

Seared Tofu with Gingered Vegetables
Ingredients:

1 pound reduced-fat extra firm tofu
1 (3 1/2-ounce) bag boil-in-bag long-grain rice
3/4 tsp. salt, divided
1 tbsp. dark sesame oil, divided
1 tbsp. bottled minced garlic
1 tbsp. bottled ground fresh ginger
1 large red bell pepper, thinly sliced
1 cup sliced green onions, divided
2 tbsp. rice vinegar
1 tbsp. low-sodium soy sauce
Cooking spray
1/4 tsp. freshly ground black pepper
1 tbsp. sesame seeds, toasted
1 cup radish sprouts

Directions:
Place tofu on several layers of paper towels; let stand 10 minutes. Cut tofu into 1-inch cubes.

Prepare rice according to package directions, omitting salt and fat. Add 1/4 teaspoon salt to rice; fluff with a fork.

Heat 2 teaspoons oil in a large nonstick skillet over medium-high heat. Add garlic, ginger, and bell pepper to pan; sauté for 3 minutes. Stir in 3/4 cup onions, vinegar, and soy sauce; cook for 30 seconds. Remove from pan. Wipe skillet with paper towels; recoat pan with cooking spray.

Place pan over medium-high heat. Sprinkle tofu with remaining 1/2 teaspoon salt and black pepper. Add tofu to pan; cook 8 minutes or until golden, turning to brown on all sides. Return bell pepper mixture to pan and cook 1 minute or until thoroughly heated. Drizzle tofu mixture with remaining 1 teaspoon oil; top with sesame seeds. Serve tofu mixture with rice; top with sprouts and remaining 1/4 cup onions.

Week 1, Day 6
Breakfast
Sweet Morning Potato

Lunch

Mediterranean Pita
1 cup carrot sticks
1 tbsp. vegan dressing

Snack
1 cup unsweetened applesauce
1 serving pretzels

Dinner
¼ of Zucchini Lasagna
1 cup roasted cauliflower in 1 tbsp butter

Snack
½ cup trail mix (1/8 cup sunflower seeds, 1/8 cup dried cranberries, 1/8 cup rice puffs, 1/8 cup raisins)

Nutrition Content For The Day
Calories: 1729
Fat: 56 g, 9 g saturated
Protein: 54.2 g
Potassium: 2685 mg
Phosphorus: 371 mg

Sweet Morning Potato
Serves 1
Ingredients:
1 sweet potato or yam, scrubbed and dried
6 ounces vanilla soy yogurt
2 tbsp. chopped walnuts

Directions:
Heat the oven to 375°F. Pierce the sweet potato several times with the tines of a fork. Place the sweet potato inside a loose nest of foil. Bake until tender when pierced with the tip of a paring knife, 40 to 50 minutes. Remove them from the oven and let them cool enough to handle.

Mediterranean Pita
Ingredients:
1 medium pita

3 tbsp. Babaghanoush spread
¼ cup chopped cucumber
1 tbsp. diced red onion
¼ cup romaine lettuce

Directions: Fill pita with all ingredients and eat.

Zucchini Lasagna

Ingredients:
3 cloves garlic
1/2 onion
2 tbsp. olive oil
2 tsp. black pepper
28 oz. can crushed tomatoes
1 can pinto beans
2 tbsp. chopped fresh basil
3 medium zucchini, sliced 1/8" thick

Directions:
Add olive oil to the pan and saute garlic and onions about 2 minutes. Add tomatoes, basil, salt and pepper. Simmer on low for at least 30-40 minutes, covered. Add can of drained and rinsed pinto beans.

Meanwhile, slice zucchini into 1/8" thick slices. On a gas grill or grill pan, grill zucchini on each side, until cooked, about 1-2 minutes per side. Place on paper towels to soak any excess moisture. Preheat oven to 350°.

In a 9x12 casserole spread some sauce on the bottom and layer the zucchini to cover. and repeat the process until all your ingredients are used up. Bake 45 minutes covered at 375°, then uncovered 15 minutes.

Let stand about 5 - 10 minutes before serving.

Week 1, Day 7
Breakfast
1 Peanut Butter Banana Smoothie

Lunch

Gourmet Almond Butter and Jelly Sandwich
1 cup celery and carrot strips
2 tbsp. Italian dressing

Snack
1 cup roasted chickpeas in olive oil

Dinner
2 cups Lentil, Kale and Potato Soup
2 sliced low-carb bread with 1 tablespoon butter

Snack
1 cup grapes
½ cup vegan light ice cream

Nutrition Content for the Day
Calories: 1790
Fat: 63 g, 7 g saturated
Protein: 59 g
Potassium: 2280 mg
Phosphorus: 553 mg

Peanut Butter Banana Smoothie
Ingredients:
1 small banana
2 tbsp. peanut butter
12 oz rice milk
Ice

Directions: Blend all ingredients until smooth. Serve immediately.

Gourmet Almond Butter and Jelly Sandwich
Ingredients:
2 slices low-carb bread
2 tbsp. almond butter
½ thinly sliced apple
2 tbsp. jelly

Lentil, Kale and Potato Soup

Serves 4
Ingredients
1 tbsp. olive oil
1 medium onion, diced
2 stalks of celery, diced
2 large carrots, diced
1 cup dry lentils
4 cups vegetables broth
½ cup water
½ tsp. garlic powder
¼ tsp. cumin
¼ tsp. coriander
1 large potato, diced
½ bunch kale, ribs removed and chopped finely
2 tsp. red wine vinegar

Directions:
Heat olive oil in a heavy-bottomed pot over medium heat. Add onion, celery, and carrots and sauté until softened, about ten minutes.

Add lentils, broth, water, salt, garlic, cumin, and coriander. Stir together and bring to a boil. Once soup has reached a boil, reduce heat to low and simmer, covered for 20 minutes.

Add chopped potatoes and simmer, covered for 15 more minutes or until potatoes are fork tender.

Add kale and simmer, covered for 5 more minutes, or until kale is wilted.

Remove from heat and stir in red wine vinegar. Season to taste with salt and pepper.

Week 2, Day 1

<u>**Breakfast**</u>
5 Minute Vegan Breakfast Smoothie

<u>**Lunch**</u>
2 cups Italian Vegetable Soup
1-5 inch breadstick

Snack
1 medium apple

Dinner
½ Stuffed Winter Squash
1 cup roasted green beans

Snack
1 cup sliced celery
2 tbsp. peanut butter

Nutrition Content For The Day
Calories: 1628
Fat: 62.6 g, 17.6 g saturated
Carbohydrates: 248 g
Protein: 48 g
Potassium: 2805 mg
Phosphorus: 521.5 mg

5-Minute Vegan Breakfast Smoothie
Serves 1
Ingredients:
1 cup almond milk
1 ripe banana, sliced
1 cup frozen fruit medley (strawberry, mango, pineapple)
1 tbsp. coconut oil
1 tbsp. chia seeds

Directions:
Combine the almond milk, banana, frozen fruit, coconut oil, and chia seeds in a blender and purée until smooth. Pour into a glass and serve immediately.

Italian Vegetable Soup
Ingredients
2 tbsp. extra-virgin olive oil
1 medium onion, finely chopped
3 to 4 cloves garlic, minced
1 small eggplant, diced (see Note)

1 to 1 1/2 cups sliced cremini or baby bella mushrooms
1 medium zucchini, or 1 yellow summer squash
10 to 12 oz. chard, (any variety)
15 to 16 oz. can diced tomatoes (use Italian-style or fire-roasted)
1 tsp. dried oregano
1/2 tsp. dried thyme
2 cups cooked or on 15 to 16 oz. can white beans or chickpeas
1/4 cup minced fresh parsley
6 to 8 leaves fresh basil, thinly sliced

Directions:
Heat the oil in a steep-sided stir fry pan or large steep-sided skillet. Add the onion and sauté over medium-low heat until translucent. Add the garlic and continue to sauté until both are golden.
Layer the eggplant, mushrooms and squash in the pan in that order and pour in 1/2 cup water. Cover and cook over medium heat for 5 minutes.

Meanwhile, strip or cut the chard leaves away from the stems. Slice the stems thinly and cut the leaves into narrow ribbons. Add the tomatoes, oregano, and thyme, and give everything a good stir. Stir in the chard and beans.
Cover and continue to simmer over low heat for 5 to 10 minutes, or until the vegetables are just tender. Stir-in basil and parsley and serve.

Savory Stuffed Winter Squash
Ingredients:
3 medium winter squashes
2 tbsp. milled chia seeds
2 1/3 cups water
1 cup kasha (buckwheat groats)
2 tblsp. extra-virgin olive oil
2 cups fresh shiitake mushrooms, stems removed and caps sliced
1 cup leeks or onions, coarsely chopped
1 cup celery, sliced
1 cup red bell pepper, coarsely chopped
1 tbsp. fresh thyme leaves or 1 ½ tsp. dried
2 tsp. fresh sage, coarsely chopped, or 1 tsp. dried
¼ cup hemp seeds

Directions:
Place the milled chia seeds in a small bowl with 1/3 cup water; set aside and boil 2 cups water in a tea kettle.

Heat and melt the red palm oil in a 9-inch heavy skillet. Add mushrooms, leeks, celery, red bell peppers, kasha, chia mixture, and sauté mixing occasionally for 5 minutes, or until the ingredients are fragrant and well mixed. Turn off the heat.

Add the boiling water and bring the ingredients to a boil over high heat. Reduce the heat to medium low and simmer covered for 10 minutes, or until the water is absorbed. Add and stir in the thyme and sage. Taste and adjust the seasonings, if desired. Let cool briefly and serve stuffed into baked winter squashes such as acorn or carnival, garnished with hemp seeds.

Week 2, Day 2

Breakfast
6 oz. soy yogurt
2 tbsp. chopped almonds
½ cup diced strawberries

Lunch
1 Loaded Vegetable Salad
1 cup chopped pineapple

Snack
1 cup raspberries

Dinner
2 Avocado Quesadillas
1 cup bell pepper strips with 1 tbsp. dressing

Snack
¼ cup dry roasted edamame

Nutrition Content For The Day
Calories: 1719
Fat: 63.9 g, 15. 6 g saturated
Carbohydrates: 266 g
Protein: 48.5 g

Potassium: 2634 mg
Phosphorus: 511.7 mg

Loaded Vegetable Salad
Ingredients:
2 cups baby spinach
½ cup green peas
½ cup chopped bell peppers
½ cup diced cucumbers
1 tbsp. olive oil
1 tbsp. balsamic vinegar

Directions: Toss all vegetables with oil and vinegar and serve.

Avocado Quesadillas
Serves: 3
Ingredients:
6 soft taco-size (8-inch) flour tortillas
1 large firm ripe avocado, finely diced
2 to 3 scallions, minced
1 cup black beans
¼ cup salsa
Shredded lettuce for garnish

Directions:
Spread the tortillas out flat and divide the diced avocado, beans, and scallions among them. Arrange the filling on one half of each tortilla, leaving about a l/2-inch border near the edges. Fold each tortilla over to make a half-circle. On a hot dry griddle, cook the quesadillas on both sides until nicely golden brown (flip them carefully).

Arrange one quesadilla on each serving plate and cut in half with a sharp knife to make two wedges. Top with a bit of the salsa.

Week 2, Day 3

Breakfast
6 oz. almond milk yogurt
1 cup mixed berries (strawberries, blueberries, blackberries)

Lunch
1 Hummus and Rice Wrap
1 medium corn on the cob

Snack
½ cup dried apples
1 oz. peanuts

Dinner
2 Lentil Sloppy Joe Sandwiches
1 cup roasted asparagus
8 oz. rice milk

Snack
2 cups air popped popcorn

Nutrition Content For The Day
Calories: 1729
Fat: 62.8 g, 15 g saturated
Protein: 273 g
Potassium: 2709 mg
Phosphorus: 528.5 mg

Hummus and Rice Wrap
Servings: Makes 2 wraps
Ingredients:
Two 10-inch wraps
1/2 to 3/4 cup hummus
2 tbsp. hemp seeds, optional
1 medium tomato, thinly sliced
1/2 cup or so cooked rice
1/4 cup sun-dried tomato strips
Mixed baby greens

Directions:
Place a wrap on a plate. Spread with about 1/4 cup hummus, and sprinkle with hemp seeds, if you'd like. Arrange half of the rice down the center of the wrap. Put a big handful of leafy greens next to it on one side, and sliced tomato on the other. Sprinkle strips of the dried tomatoes here and there.

Fold two sides of the wrap over the ends of the row of rice, keeping them tucked in as you roll the wrap snugly to enclose all the ingredients.

Lentil Sloppy Joes
Makes 8 sandwiches
Ingredients:
1 1/2 cup brown lentils, rinsed and picked over
1 yellow onion, diced (about 2 1/2 cups)
1 red bell pepper, seeded and diced (about 1 1/2 cups)
1 1/2 tbsp. chili powder
2 tsp. paprika
1 1/2 tsp. ground cumin
1/8 tsp. cayenne pepper (optional)
1 (6-ounce) can no-salt-added tomato paste
2 tbsp. red wine vinegar
6 cloves garlic, minced
1 (15-ounce) can no-salt-added crushed tomatoes
8 whole wheat low-carb hamburger buns

Directions:
Place lentils in a small pot. Cover with 2 inches of water. Cover and bring to a boil, then reduce to a simmer. Cook until lentils are tender, about 30 minutes. Meanwhile, heat a large skillet over medium-high heat. Add onion and bell pepper. Cook, stirring frequently until onion is golden brown, about 5 minutes. Add chili powder, paprika, cumin, cayenne, and tomato paste. Cook, stirring constantly until spices and tomato paste are fragrant, about 2 minutes. Add vinegar and then use a wooden spoon to scrape up any bits from the bottom of the pan. Add 2 cups water, garlic, and crushed tomatoes. Reduce heat to medium-low and let sauce simmer until it thickens, at least 30 minutes.

When lentils are cooked, drain off any excess cooking liquid. Add lentils to the pan with sauce; stir well to combine. Mash some or all of the lentils using a wooden spoon. Toast hamburger buns in the oven, if desired. Ladle 1 cup of the lentil mixture on each toasted bun and serve.

Week 2, Day 4

Breakfast
2 Zucchini Raisin Muffins
1 tbsp. butter
1 cup rice milk

Lunch
2 cups Roasted Vegetable Salad
6 whole grain crackers

Snack
¼ cup dry roasted edamame, ¼ cup dried cranberries

Dinner
White Bean and Sweet Potato Burger on bun with 1 slice tomato, 1 piece lettuce, 2 tsp. mustard
Side salad (1 cup lettuce, ¼ cup tomato, ¼ cup cucumber)
2 tbsp. dressing (1 tbsp. olive oil, 1 tbsp. vinegar)

Snack
1 cup mixed berries (strawberries, blueberries, blackberries)

Nutrition Content For Day
Calories: 1673
Fat: 53.5 g, 6.4 g saturated
Carbohydrates: 258.9 g
Protein: 63 g
Potassium: 2905 mg
Phosphorus: 394.8 mg

Zucchini Raisin Muffins
Ingredients:
2 cups whole wheat pastry or light spelt flour
(or your favorite gluten-free flour blend)
1/2 cup natural granulated sugar
1 1/2 tsp. baking powder
1/2 tsp. baking soda
1/2 tsp. cinnamon
1 cup applesauce
2 tbsp. safflower oil
1/4 cup plain or vanilla rice nondairy milk

1 tsp. vanilla extract
1 cup firmly packed grated zucchini
1/2 cup raisins
1/4 cup chopped walnuts, optional
1/2 cup chocolate chips, optional

Directions:
Preheat the oven to 350 degrees F.
5 (dry) ingredients in a mixing bowl. Make a well in the center of the dry ingredients and pour in the applesauce, oil, and nondairy milk. Stir together until combined. Don't overbeat! If need be add just another splash of nondairy milk to combine wet and dry, but let it remain a stiff batter.

Stir in the zucchini, raisins, and optional walnuts and/or chocolate chips.

Divide the batter between 12 muffin tins and bake for 20 to 25 minutes, or until the tops are golden and a small knife inserted in the center of a muffin tests clean. Cool on a rack. To transport in a lunch box, place in a container that will protect the muffins from being crushed.

Roasted Vegetable Salad
Ingredients:
½ cup sliced zucchini
½ cup sliced summer squash
½ cup diced onions
½ cup sliced carrots
2 tbsp. chopped basil
1 tbsp. olive oil

Directions: Toss all vegetables together with basil and olive oil. Roast at 425 degrees for about 30 minutes until vegetables are cooked through. Mix vegetables about halfway through.

White Bean and Sweet Potato Burgers
Makes: 8-10 veggie burgers
Ingredients:
2 cups cooked white beans, drained

1 1/2 cup mashed sweet potato (can be roasted, steamed or boiled)
1 medium onion
2 cloves garlic
1/2 cup parsley
1 tsp. ground cumin
Several dashes of freshly ground black pepper
Pinch of chili powder
3/4 cup breadcrumbs
3/4 cup soy flour

Directions:
In a food processor add the onion, garlic, parsley, and white beans and pulse until beans are broken.

Add the sweet potato puree and spices and pulse a few more times.

Transfer to a big mixing bowl, add the breadcrumbs and soy flour, and mix with your hands for about 2 minutes.
Place the mixture in the refrigerator for at least 30 minutes.
Form the mixture into burger patties, place on a baking sheet, brush with olive oil, and bake in preheated oven at 180C/350F for 30 minutes, flipping once. Enjoy!

Week 2, Day 5

Breakfast
Very Berry Smoothie

Lunch
2 cups Mango Lentil Salad
1 slice bread with 2 tsp. butter

Snack
Sliced apple with 1 tblsp. almond butter

Dinner
2 Bean Burritos
½ avocado with ¼ cup chopped tomato and 2 tbsp. cilantro

Snack

1 oz. roasted almonds

Nutrition Content For The Day
Calories: 1593
Fat: 54.5 g, 5.6 g saturated
Carbohydrates: 253 g
Protein: 49 g
Potassium: 2406 mg
Phosphorus: 513.1 mg

Very Berry Smoothie
Ingredients:
12 oz rice milk
½ cup frozen blueberries
½ cup frozen strawberries
½ cup frozen raspberries

Directions: Blend all ingredients together and serve.

Mango Lentil Salad
Ingredients:
1/2 cup dry lentils (about 2 cups cooked)
2 tbsp. cold pressed extra virgin olive oil
1/2 tsp. ground coriander
1/2 tsp. ground cumin
Juice of 1 lime
1 mango, peeled and diced
1/2 red onion, chopped
2 tbsp. chopped fresh cilantro leaves, plus more for garnish

Directions:
Put the lentils in a fine strainer and pick through them, discarding any bits of stone that may be present. Rinse under cold running water. Place in a pot and cover with 3 to 4 inches of water, bring to a boil, then reduce to a simmer.

Check lentils after 15 to 20 minutes; they should have slight resistance to the tooth — you want them *al dente*. Remove from heat, drain and place under cold running water to stop the cooking process. Once cooled slightly, combine the lentils with mango and onion in a large bowl.

In a small jar or bowl, combine the olive oil, coriander, cumin, lime juice and cilantro leaves. Pour over the lentils, mango, and onion. Toss to combine. Garnish with some more cilantro leaves.

Bean Burritos
Serves: 4
Ingredients:
Filling:
1 tbsp. olive oil
1 small onion, chopped
1 clove garlic, minced
1/2 medium green bell pepper, finely diced
3 cups well-cooked pinto beans
One 4-oz. can chopped mild green chilis
2 to 4 tbsp. minced fresh cilantro, to taste
1 tsp. ground cumin

Remaining ingredients:
8 burrito-size (10- to 12-inch) flour tortillas
1 cup firmly packed cheddar-style non-dairy cheese
Salsa
Shredded lettuce for garnish
Black olives for garnish

Directions:
Heat the oil in a medium skillet. Add the onion and sauté over medium-low heat until it is translucent. Add the garlic and sauté for another minute before adding the green pepper. Continue to sauté until the onion is lightly golden. Add the pinto beans along with the remaining filling ingredients and enough liquid to keep the mixture moist. Simmer, covered, for 10 minutes.

With a mashing implement, mash about half of the beans. Make sure there is enough liquid in the mixture to form a thick, saucy base. Cook, covered, for another 5 minutes.
Spoon some of the bean mixture onto the centers of each flour tortilla. Sprinkle with some grated cheese, if desired, and top with a spoonful or so of salsa. Fold the burritos as directed in the illustration below.

Arrange 2 burritos on each dinner plate. Garnish with shredded lettuce and black olives. Pass around extra salsa. Serve at once.

Week 2, Day 6

Breakfast
English muffin with 2 tbsp. almond butter
1 cup rice milk

Lunch
2 cups Vegan Chili
1 cup rice milk

Snack
1 cup Kale Chips

Dinner
2 cups Vegetable Chow Mein
1 cup roasted sugar snap peas

Snack
1 medium peach
2 cups air popped popcorn

Nutrition Content For The Day
Calories: 1698
Fat: 57 g, 6 g saturated
Carbohydrates: 268 g
Protein: 56 g
Potassium: 2482 mg
Phosphorus: 588 mg

Vegan Chili
Serves: 6 to 8
Ingredients:
1 tbsp. olive oil
2 medium onions, finely chopped
2 cloves garlic, minced
1 large green bell pepper, finely chopped

4 cups cooked pinto or pink beans (about 1 2/3 cups raw, or two 16-oz. cans, drained and rinsed)
28-oz. can crushed tomatoes
1 1/2 cups cooked fresh or thawed frozen corn kernels
1 to 2 fresh hot chili peppers, seeded and minced, or
4-oz. can mild or hot chopped green chiles
1 tsp. dried oregano
2 to 3 tsp. good-quality chili powder, more or less to taste
1 tsp. ground cumin

Directions:
Heat the oil in a large soup pot. Add the onion and garlic and sauté over medium heat until the onion is golden.

Add the remaining ingredients except the salt. Simmer gently, covered, for 30 minutes, stirring occasionally. If the consistency seems too dense, add 1/2 cup of water at a time, until the consistency is just the way you like it (though let it stay nice and thick).

Season gently with salt and adjust the other seasonings. If time allows, let stand for an hour or so off the heat, then heat through as needed before serving. Serve in bowls.

Kale Chips
Ingredients:
1 head of kale, torn into bite sized pieces
2 tbsp. olive oil
½ tsp. onion powder
½ tsp. garlic powder

Directions: Mix all ingredients well and roast at 400 degrees until kale chips are crispy.

Vegetable Chow Mein
Serves: 4 to 6
Ingredients:
12 oz. wide Chinese wheat noodles
2 tbsp. olive or peanut oil
1 large onion, quartered and sliced
3 large stalks celery or bok choy, sliced on a diagonal

1 medium bunch broccoli, cut into bite-sized florets and stems
1 red bell pepper, cut into narrow strips
8-oz. fresh mung bean sprouts
15-oz. can straw mushrooms, liquid reserved
6- or 8-oz. can sliced water chestnuts, liquid reserved
Liquid from straw mushrooms and water chestnuts (about 1 to 1 1/4 cups)
2 tbsp. arrowroot or cornstarch
2 tbsp. reduced-sodium soy sauce

Directions:
Cook the noodles in plenty of rapidly simmering water until just tender, then drain.

Meanwhile, heat the oil in a stir-fry pan. Add the onion and stir-fry over medium heat until translucent.

Add the celery, broccoli, and bell pepper, and stir-fry over medium-high heat until all are just tender-crisp. Stir in the sprouts, mushrooms, and water chestnuts, and continue to cook until everything is well heated through.

In a small bowl, combine 1/4 cup of the reserved liquid from canned vegetables with the cornstarch and stir until dissolved. Stir in the remaining liquid and the soy sauce. Pour the sauce into the pan and cook just until it has thickened.

Remove from the heat and gently stir the cooked noodles together with the vegetables. Serve at once, passing around extra soy sauce, if desired.

Week 2, Day 7

Breakfast
1 serving Chia Breakfast Bowl

Lunch
2 cups Rice and Asparagus Salad
1 cup raw baby carrots

Snack

½ cup dried apples
¼ cup peanuts

Dinner
Vegan Greek Salad
Small pita toasted

Snack
1 medium pear

Nutrition Content For Day
Calories: 1697
Fat: 62.8 g, 6.3 g saturated
Carbohydrates:254 g
Protein: 50.4 g
Potassium: 2605 mg
Phosphorus: 531.3 mg

Chia Breakfast Bowl
Serves: 2
Ingredients:
¼ cup whole chia seeds
2 cups unsweetened nondairy milk of your choice
2 tbsp. pure maple syrup
1 tsp. vanilla extract
Toppings:
Fresh fruit of your choice (mangos, bananas, berries, kiwi, pineapple, etc.)
2 tbsp. almonds

Directions:
Combine the chia seeds, nondairy milk, syrup, and vanilla extract in a bowl and stir together. Let stand for about a half hour, then whisk together to prevent the seeds from clumping. Transfer to an air-tight container, cover and refrigerate overnight.In the morning, divide between two bowls, and serve with toppings of your choice.

Rice and Asparagus Salad
Serves 6
Ingredients:

1 cup raw rice, any color, or a combination, rinsed
10- to 12-oz. fresh slender asparagus
1 medium red bell pepper, diced
1/4 cup finely chopped fresh parsley, or more, to taste
2 to 3 scallions, finely chopped
Several fresh mint leaves, to taste, thinly sliced, optional
2 tbsp. extra-virgin olive oil
Juice of 1 lime, or more, to taste
Salt and freshly ground pepper to taste
Lime wedges for serving, optional

Directions:
Combine the rice with 2 cups water in a small saucepan. Bring to a gentle boil, then lower the heat, cover, and simmer until the water is absorbed, about 15 minutes. If you'd like a more tender grain, add 1/2 cup additional water and continue to simmer until the water is absorbed. Allow to cool to room temperature.

Meanwhile, scrape the bottom halves of the asparagus spears if need be. If fresh and tender, you can skip this step. Cut the asparagus into 1- to 2-inch pieces. Place in a skillet with just enough water to keep the bottom moist. Cover and steam over medium heat just until bright green and tender-crisp. Transfer the asparagus to a colander and rinse with water until it's at room temperature.

Combine with the rice and asparagus with the remaining ingredients in a serving bowl and mix well. Let stand for a few minutes, then serve. Pass around extra wedges of lime, if you'd like.

Vegan Greek Salad
Ingredients:
2 cups romaine lettuce
1 chopped small tomato
½ cup chopped cucumber
2 tbsp. kalamata olives
1/3 cup chickpeas (drained and rinsed)
¼ cup beets
3 tbsp. Greek dressing

Directions: Mix all ingredients together and serve

The Academy of Nutrition and Dietetics Kidney Disease Diet

The Academy of Nutrition and Dietetics is an organization of food and nutrition professionals founded in Cleveland, Ohio, in 1917, by a group of women dedicated to helping the government conserve food and improve the public's health and nutrition during World War I.

Today, the Academy credentializes practitioners as registered dietitian, dietetic technicians and other dietetics professionals holding undergraduate and advanced degrees; It is committed to improving the nation's health and advancing the profession of dietetics through research, education and advocacy.

Dietetic practitioners work in health care systems, home health care, food service, business, research and educational organizations, as well as in private practice. Community-based dietetic practitioners provide health promotion, disease prevention and wellness services.

The major difference of dietitians and other nutrition professionals is they follow the recommendations set forth by the Academy.

These diet recommendations are very helpful for kidney disease, but only comprise one dietary approach taught to their students.

They do not take into account other diet approaches supported by science. They also don't recognize the harmful effects of refined sugar. However, the Academy's kidney diet is more manageable for many people with kidney disease, due to its larger variety of foods. It still provides plenty of benefits for kidney disease.

Overview of Diet

The Dietetic approach to dealing with Chronic Kidney Disease is centered around achieving optimal balance of protein, sodium and potassium, doing so through the foods that you eat. It has more of a focus on animal products, as opposed to the low protein and vegetarian diet.

There are many benefits that can be reaped from the diet alone and there are a lot of steps you can implement into your diet to achieve better kidney health right away.

Let's go forward and briefly touch upon each cornerstone of the Academy's diet, so you will have a good understanding of how it will help chronic kidney disease. You can check with your insurance to see what dietitians may be in your plan, if you are interested in working with this type of professional.

Protein

Protein is responsible for a lot of the body's functions. It most notably helps to keep every cell in working order, repairing and building any elements that are worn down and even supplying energy in some instances. It's found abundantly in animal food sources (various meats, poultry, fish, milk and eggs), along with beans, seeds and nuts.

That being said, protein is a necessary part of any diet and the Academy of Dietetics does include more recipes, which incorporate a moderate amount of animal protein

How can you tell how much protein you need daily? Undoubtedly, each person's needs vary based on age, sex and overall general health. The Recommended Dietary Allowance (RDA) for protein in healthy adults is 0.8 grams of protein per kilogram of desirable body weight a day. So, for a 150 pound person (divide by 2.2 to get 68 kilograms then multiply by 0.8), that is 55 grams of protein a day. For someone who weighs 120 pounds, that would be 44 grams of protein a day.

Animal sources of protein are termed "complete" or "high quality" as they provide all the essential amino acids (the building blocks of protein). Animal sources of protein can vary in their amount of fat, with fatty cuts of red meat and whole-milk dairy products and eggs being the highest in saturated fat, which are less heart-healthy. Fish, poultry, and low-fat or fat-free dairy products are lower in saturated fat. An "incomplete" or "lower quality" protein source is one that is low in one or more of the essential amino acids. Plant sources such as beans, lentils, nuts, peanut butter, seeds and whole grains are examples of incomplete proteins.

The good news is that if you eat a combination of these incomplete proteins in the same day, they can provide adequate amounts of all the essential amino acids. Vegetarians can meet their protein needs with careful planning. For example, combining red beans and rice or peanut butter on whole grain bread together make a complete protein. Another bonus with plant proteins is that they are low in saturated fat and high in fiber.

Examples of the amount of protein in the typical serving sizes of the major protein foods:

- 1 whole egg or 1/4 cup frozen egg substitute = 7 grams
- 3 ounces cooked meat (size of a deck of cards) = 21–24 grams (leaner meats are higher in protein per oz.)
- 8 ounces milk (whole, 2%, skim, soy) = 8 grams
- 8 ounces yogurt or 1 ounce cheese = 8 grams
- 1 cup cooked beans (navy, pinto, kidney, black-eyed peas, split peas) = 14–16 grams
- 1 ounce of dry roasted peanuts = 7 grams

Total protein from above sources = 65–70 grams

Sodium

Sodium is commonly found in many packaged, processed foods as a seasoning and as a preservative. It's almost impossible to avoid an abundance of salt in the common American diet but holding back on salt is important according to the Academy of Dietetics. It's best to avoid sodium and use alternative salt-free seasonings and to always read food labels and make sure you're picking the lowest sodium option available. Sodium intake should be kept at 1500-2000mg per day.

Potassium

Potassium is another mineral that is important to monitor in the Dietetic Diet. It can help regulate the heart beat and enables your muscles to function more smoothly. A lower potassium diet consists of 2400 mg per day. It's important to space out the presence of higher potassium vegetables as a part of a larger meal that incorporates other kidney-friendlier foods. The monitoring of potassium levels also coincides with being careful of which seasonings you use in your meal preparation, as even many salt-substitutes contain high levels of potassium.

Phosphorus

Your kidneys primarily help to maintain phosphorous balance in the body. When kidney function is less than optimal, phosphorous can build up in the body causing calcium to control the balance of phosphorus in the body. When phosphorus builds up in the body, it can result in calcium being released from the bones. This leads to a weakening of the bones that can be very painful and put you at increased risk of breaks and fractures. An overabundance of phosphorus in the blood has also been linked to heart disease.

The Academy of Nutrition and Dietetics Food List

Kidney Friendly Foods

Fruits

Apple (1 small)	Apple sauce	Berries (all types)
Cherries	Fig (1 large)	Fruit cocktail
Grapes (17 small)	Grapefruit (1/2 large)	Lemon/Lime (1 medium)
Peach (canned, fresh nectar)	Pear	Pineapple (canned, fresh)
Plum	Raspberries	Tangerine/Clementine (1 small)
Watermelon (1/2 cup)		

Vegetables

Alfalfa sprouts	Asparagus	Bamboo shoots (canned)
Beans: green or yellow (cooked)	Cabbage	Carrots (canned or cooked)
Cauliflower (cooked)	Celery (8" stalk)	Corn (or one 6" ear)
Cucumber	Eggplant	Leeks
Lettuce	Mustard greens (cooked)	Okra (cooked)
Onions	Peppers: green, red, jalapeño or chili (cooked)	Radishes (raw)
Spinach (raw)	Turnip greens	Turnips (cooked)

Water chestnuts (canned)	Zucchini	Snap Peas
Shallots	Garlic	Broccoli

Bread, Cereals and Grain Products

Angel food cake	Animal crackers or vanilla wafers	Bagel
Bread: French, Italian, light rye, sourdough, white	Bun (sandwich)	Cake: plain (2x2 inch), Homemade
Cereals ready-to-eat, except bran, oat-based, or whole wheat	Cooked cereals, except oats or instant	Cookies: apple, berry, butter, lemon, shortbread, sugar
Crackers, unsalted (6)	Danish pastry or sweet roll (small)	Donut, cake (1)
Dinner or hard roll (small)	English muffin (1/2)	Flour tortilla (6-inch)
Graham crackers (3 squares)	Melba toast	Muffin (small)
Pasta: macaroni, noodles, spaghetti	Pita pocket	Popcorn, plain, unsalted
Pretzels, unsalted	Rice, white	Roll, white
Bulgur Wheat	Couscous	Rice cakes
White flour	Rice Pilaf	

Milk Substitutes & Beverages

Almond milk	Rice milk, un-enriched	Frozen non-dairy desserts
Fruit Ices	Popsicles	Snow Cones
Apple juice	Apricot nectar	Cranberry juice cocktail
Grape juice	Grapefruit juice	Peach Nectar
Lemon/Lime Juice	Pineapple Juice	Limeade

Mello Yello	Sprite	7UP
Ginger Ale	Club Soda	Coffee Mate
Non-enriched Soy Milk	Non-dairy Frozen Whipped Topping	

Meats/Proteins

Beef, lean	Chicken, skinless	Egg or egg whites
Lamb	Pork, lean or pork loin	Turkey, skinless
Veal	Wild Game	Beans (such as black or kidney)
Peas (such as split peas)	Fish	Turkey Bacon (low salt)
Shellfish	Lentils	Chickpea/Hummus
Reduced Sodium Broths		

Oils/Fats/Dairy/Misc.

Sesame Seed Oil	Flax Seed Oil	Canola Oil
Coconut Oil	Walnut Oil	Extra Virgin Olive Oil
Any Cooking Oils Can Be Used	Cream Cheese, (1-2 tbsp limit per day)	Mayonnaise
Parmesan Cheese	Skim Ricotta Cheese	Light Sour Cream
Low Fat Yogurt	Marshmallow	Butter, unsalted

Vinegars, Salt, Seasonings and Condiments

Vinegars
All vinegars are acceptable with kidney disease; make sure no salt is added.

Salt, Seasonings and Condiments
Avoid table salt and any seasonings that have the word "salt or sodium," and avoid salt substitutes (they contain potassium) and any seasonings with potassium. Purchase the lowest sodium foods you can and don't add salt to any foods. Most other seasonings are acceptable. Keep sodium intake to 1500-2000mg per day.

List of Seasonings and Condiments
Allspice, basil, bay leaf, caraway seed, chives, cilantro, cinnamon, cloves, cumin, curry, dill, extracts (almond, lemon, lime, maple, orange, peppermint, vanilla, walnut), fennel, garlic powder, ginger, horseradish (root), lemon juice, low sodium hot sauce like Tabasco®, mustard, Mrs. Dash®, nutmeg, onion powder or flakes, oregano, paprika, parsley flakes, pepper (ground), pimentos, poppy seed, rosemary, saffron, sage, savory, sesame seeds, tarragon, thyme, turmeric, vegan mayo (not made with soy, check protein content).

Salad Dressings
It is best to make your own with oil, vinegar, spices and vegan mayo. Some Russian, French, and Ranch dressings have low potassium and protein levels and can be consumed.

Sweeteners
Stevia is a great natural sweetener and small amounts of maple syrup and honey are also allowed. Jams and jellies that are low-sugar and made from the list of kidney-friendly fruits are also safe to consume in moderate amounts.

Fruits, Vegetables, Whole Grains & Other Foods Not Listed

For the most part other foods not listed on the program should be avoided or used in small amounts and not often.

If you know your levels of potassium and they are in the lower to middle ranges you can consume some fruits and vegetables that are not listed in small quantities.

Generally, the Academy's kidney disease diet does not include whole grains due to their higher phosphorus content. If you know your phosphorous levels and they are in the low to middle range, you can consume small quantities of whole grains, but not often.

The Academy of Nutrition and Dietetics 'MyPlate' Method

Use this as a guide for choosing portion size and balancing nutrients

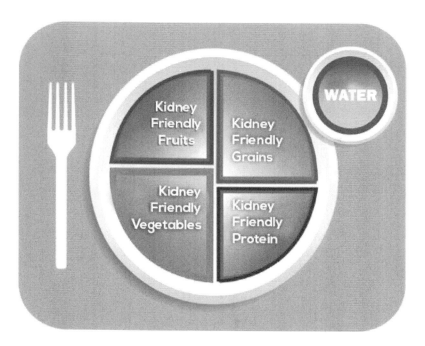

The Academy of Nutrition and Dietetics Sample Menu Plan

Week 1, Day 1

Breakfast
1 plain bagel toasted with 1 tsp. unsalted butter & 1 T apple butter
1 cup rice milk
2 slices low sodium turkey bacon
1 medium peach

Lunch
Italian Grilled Chicken Sandwich
Apple – 1 small to moderate size

Snack
1 rice cake

Dinner
1 to 2 cups *Lemon Rice*
2 ounces baked tilapia
½ cup steamed green beans
You can add 2 to 3 tablespoons of olive oil to any rice dish

Snack
1 cup grapes

Nutrition Content For Day
Calories: 1522
Fat: 46 g, 10 g saturated
Carbohydrates: 264 g
Protein: 59 g
Potassium: 1899 mg
Phosphorus: 668 mg
Sodium: 1056 mg

Recipes For The Day
Italian Grilled Chicken Sandwich
Ingredients:
2 slices white bread
1 tbsp olive oil
3 oz grilled chicken
1 slice eggplant
1 slice roasted pepper
1 to 2 slices of salad leaves

Directions:
Place 1 slice of bread on heated, oiled skillet. Layer oil, grilled chicken, eggplant, roasted pepper, and salad leaves. Top with 2nd slice of bread. Grill until golden brown.

Spicy Gold Rice
Ingredients:
2 ½ tbsp. olive oil
1 small onion, chopped
1 medium jalapeno pepper, minced
2 T. lemon juice
¼ tsp. lemon zest
1 cup long grain rice
low-sodium chicken stock or water for rice
1 bay leaf

Directions:
In a saucepan, heat oil over medium low heat. Add the onion, pepper and stir until onion is translucent, about 6 to 8 minutes.

Mix in lemon juice and zest. Add the rice and stir for 2 minutes to coat the rice with the spice mix. Add stock or water, bring to boil, reduce heat to low, cover and cook until all liquid is absorbed.

Week 1, Day 2
Breakfast
2 pancakes
2 tablespoon butter
1 ½ tablespoon maple syrup

Snack
10 *Apple Rings*
1 cup rice milk

Lunch
1 to 1 ½ cup *Sunny Penne*
2 oz. baked lean pork chop
1 slice bread with 1 tsp. butter

Snack
1 small plum
1 oz pretzels, no salt

Dinner
1 to 2 cup *Steak (not to be eaten often)* with *Cauliflower Mash*
1 cup grapes

Snack
1 cup baby carrots with simple vinaigrette

Nutrition Content For Day
Calories: 1801
Fat: 61 g, 23 g saturated
Carbohydrates: 230 g
Protein: 61 g
Potassium: 2366 mg
Phosphorus: 544 mg
Sodium: 1834 mg

Recipes For The Day
Oven Dried Apples
Ingredients:
Apples, as many as desired
A few tbsp. fresh lemon juice
A pinch or two of Stevia™ (optional)

Directions:
Preheat the oven to 150 degrees. Core the apples and slice them into ½ inch rings. Soak in a bowl of water with the lemon juice for 15 minutes, and add the stevia if using. Drain, and lay in a single layer on top of cooling racks positioned on top of a baking sheet.

Place in the oven and bake for a couple of hours, depending really on whether you want crispy apple chips or chewy dried apples. You may want to flip the rings every now and then to cook them evenly, and keep in mind to check them individually as some of them may be done before others.

Sunny Penne
Ingredients:
3 medium carrots, peeled and thinly sliced
4 small zucchini, thinly sliced
¼ cup snap peas
½ small onion, sliced thin
1 red bell pepper, sliced thin
2 medium garlic cloves
1 tbsp. dried tarragon
4 tbsp. olive oil
1 tsp. white wine vinegar
12 oz. of dry penne pasta

Directions:
Bring medium saucepan of water to a boil. Put carrots and zucchini in the water for 2 minutes. Add the peas and cook for 1 minute longer. Drain well, place in a large bowl and add the pepper, onion, garlic, tarragon, oil, vinegar.

Cook pasta according to package direction. Drain when cooked, and top with sauce.

Steak with Cauliflower Mash
(Serves 4)
Ingredients:
1 tbsp butter
6 minced garlic cloves
2 beef tenderloin medallions
6 cups cauliflower florets
3 oz reduced fat cream cheese
1 tbsp grated parmesan cheese

Directions:
Sear beef on both sides in hot skillet. Top with butter and garlic. Continue cooking in oven until desired doneness.

Steam cauliflower for 10 minutes.

Combine cauliflower with cream cheese in food processor, pulsing until smooth. Remove from food processor and blend in parmesan cheese.

Week 1, Day 3
Breakfast
1 slice Strawberry *French Toast*
You can add 1 tablespoons butter
1 to 2 tablespoons maple syrup
2 scrambled eggs

Lunch
Easy Salmon Cakes
1 slice bread with 1 tsp. butter

Snack
1 cup pineapple
¾ cup corn Chex
¼ to ½ cup rice milk

Dinner
2 cups *Quick Pasta with Broccoli*
2 oz baked chicken

Snack
1 cup raspberries

Nutrition Content For Day
Calories: 1765
Fat: 70 g, 28 g saturated
Carbohydrates: 216 g
Protein: 68 g
Potassium: 1692 mg
Phosphorus: 729 mg
Sodium: 1739 mg

Recipes For The Day
Strawberry French Toast
Ingredients:
2 slices bread
1/2 cup rice milk
1/4 tsp. lemon juice
1 tsp. olive oil
½ tsp. vanilla extract
¼ cup sliced strawberries

Directions:
In a small mixing bowl, whisk together the rice milk and lemon juice, set aside. Heat oil in skillet. Dredge bread slices in milk mixture. Place 1 slice in skillet. Top with strawberries. Top with remaining slice. Cook on both sides until golden brown.

Easy Salmon Cakes
Ingredients:
1 ½ cups cooked salmon flaked with fork
2 tsp old bay seasoning
1/3 cup egg substitute
2 tbsp mayonnaise
¾ cup panko bread crumbs
1 small, finely chopped green pepper
2 tbsp fresh chives, chopped
1 tsp lemon juice
Canola oil for frying

Directions:
Combine all ingredients in large bowl.
Form mixture into 6-8 small patties.
Place patties on oiled griddle over medium heat.
Cook 3 minutes on each side until golden brown, then flip and cook additional 3 minutes or until other side is golden brown as well. Serve with lemon and tartar sauce.

Quick Pasta with Broccoli
Ingredients:
2 cup small broccoli florets

½ cup butter
2 tbsp. dried basil
2 tbsp. dried parsley
1 small clove garlic, minced
8 oz. of dry pasta of choice

Directions:
Cut broccoli tops into small florets. In a bowl combine butter, basil, parsley, garlicup Mix ingredients well. In a saucepan, bring 4 cups of water to a boil. Add the broccoli to boiling water and cook until tender. Drain and place in a bowl, add herb butter and toss coating the broccoli.

Cook pasta according to package directions. Drain well when cooked and top with broccoli and herb butter.

Week 1, Day 4
Breakfast
1 cup Cream of Wheat hot cereal, made with rice milk
1 cup watermelon

Snack
2 plums
3 cup unsalted popcorn

Lunch
2 cups *Chicken and Grape Salad*

Snack
1 cup celery sticks with dipping sauce such as low sodium salad dressings

Dinner
1-2 cups *Fancy Rigatoni*
2 oz. *Herb Crusted Pork Tenderloins*

Snack
4 graham cracker squares
1 cup strawberries with low fat cream cheese

Nutrition Content For Day
Calories: 1026

Fat: 34 g, 7 g saturated
Carbohydrates: 137 g
Protein: 46 g
Potassium: 1885 mg
Phosphorus: 620 mg
Sodium: 693 mg

Recipes For The Day
Chicken and Grape Salad
(Serves 6)
Ingredients:
1 diced apple
1 lb rotelle pasta
½ cup seedless grapes
1 cup sliced cooked chicken
Dressing:
½ cup mayonnaise
2 tbsp sriracha hot sauce
¼ cup light sour cream

Directions:
Combine dressing ingredients in large bowl and mix well.
Add cooked pasta and mix well.
Add grapes and apples and mix well.
Transfer to serving plates and top with sliced chicken.

Fancy Rigatoni
(Serves 4)
Ingredients:
3 cups cooked rigatoni
8 oz. chicken breast
2 cloves garlic chopped
2 tbsp canola oil
½ cup chopped green onions
½ cup chopped red pepper
¼ tsp cayenne pepper
½ cup white wine
1 cup salt-free chicken broth
Bunch fresh basil torn into pieces
Bunch fresh parsley chopped fine
Paprika to taste

Directions:
Sauté garlic in oil in large skillet.
Cut chicken into strips.
Brown with garlic for 5 minutes.
Add remaining ingredients and simmer for 20 min. covered.
Remove from heat and toss in cooked pasta and herbs.
Serve with paprika sprinkled on top.

Herb Crusted Pork Tenderloins
(Serves 6)
Ingredients:
4 lb. boneless pork loin untrimmed
2 tbsp olive oil
4 cloves garlic, minced
1 tsp dried thyme
1 tsp dried basil
1 tsp dried rosemary

Directions:
Pre-heat oven to 450.
Place pork loin on a rack in a roasting pan.
Combine the remaining ingredients in small bowl Rub pork loin with paste.
Roast pork for 30 minutes
Reduce heat to 375 degrees and roast for an additional hour or until internal temp reached 160.
Allow to sit for 20 min. before carving

Week 1, Day 5
Breakfast
4 ounces of low fat yogurt
1 croissant with jam or butter
1 cup blackberries

Lunch
Tropical Chicken Salad

Snack
1 apple
10 corn chips (unsalted)

Dinner
1 to 2 c *Sautéed Vegetables and Noodles*
2 ounces grilled salmon

Snack
3 cups unsalted popcorn

Nutrition Content For Day
Calories: 1542
Fat: 60 g, 16 g saturated
Carbohydrates: 153 g
Protein: 68 g
Potassium: 1904 mg
Phosphorus: 798 mg
Sodium: 1084 mg

Tropical Chicken Salad
(Serves 4)
Ingredients:
½ cup diced celery
1 ½ cup shredded cooked chicken
1 cup peeled and diced apples
1 cup drained unsweetened pineapple chunks
½ cup seedless grapes
1 cup diced pears
½ tsp sugar
2 tbsp lemon juice
½ cup mayonnaise
Dash hot sauce
1 tsp black pepper
Paprika for garnish

Directions:
In large bowl, combine sugar, juice, mayonnaise, hot sauce and pepper.
Mix together remaining ingredients in separate bowl.
Add dressing to fruit and chicken, combining well.
Serve on bed of lettuce and sprinkle with paprika.

Sautéed Vegetables and Noodles
(Serves 4)
Ingredients:
1 tbsp olive oil
¼ cup diced red onion
3 minced garlic cloves
1 cup fresh green beans julienned
1 cup carrots julienned with mandolin
2 cups cooked spaghetti
Pinch of Saffron

Directions:
In a hot, oiled skillet cook onions and garlic for 2 minutes.
Add saffron.
Add vegetables and stir, cooking for around 3 min.
Add noodles and pepper, tossing until well-combined.

Week 1, Day 6
Breakfast
Strawberry Smoothie
1 roll with butter
1 boiled egg

Lunch
1 to 1 ½ cups of *Boiled Vegetables* over
1 to 2 cups of rice
2 oz. grilled steak (not to be eaten often)

Snack
5 to 10 pretzels (unsalted)
2 celery stalks with 1 tablespoons salad dressing for dipping

Dinner
1 to 2 cups *Linguine with Garlic, Oil, Peppers and Chicken*

Snack
1 cup blueberries
¾ cup of corn flakes
½ to 1 cup rice

Nutrition Content For Day
Calories: 1688
Fat: 44 g, 11 g saturated

Carbohydrates: 256 g
Protein: 39.2 g
Potassium: 1808 mg
Phosphorus: 768 mg
Sodium: 1631 mg

Recipes For The Day
Strawberry Smoothie
Ingredients:
1 cup strawberries
12 to 14 oz. of rice milk
4 oz. low fat yogurt
1 tsp. of vanilla extract

Directions:
Place all in a blender and combine until smooth.
You can add honey, essential amino acid powder, acacia fiber, and oils, especially fish and flaxseed.

Directions:
Blend ingredients until a smooth consistency. Adjust ingredient doses to desired amounts.

Boiled Vegetables
Directions:
1 to 2 cup of kidney-friendly vegetables (found on pg. 100). Boil vegetables till tender or as desired. Strain vegetables and season to taste. Drizzle 1 to 2 tbsps. of olive oil over vegetables.

Linguine with Garlic and Oil
Ingredients:
1 lb. (16 oz.) of linguine
½ cup olive oil
1 cup red pepper, sliced
½ cup onion, chopped
3 to 5 cloves garlic (sliced)
1 pinch dried chili pepper flakes
2 tbsp. dried parsley
1 tsp. fresh ground black pepper
1 tbsp. grated parmesan cheese
1 pound grilled chicken

Directions:
Cook linguine following the package directions. Sauté sliced garlic cloves (add more garlic, to taste), peppers, and onions in walnut oil over medium heat until tender. Remove garlic and set aside. Add dry pepper flakes, cook for an additional minute. Add parsley, cook 1 minute. Add cooked linguine, toss in garlic, arrange on serving platter, and sprinkle with black pepper and grated cheese. Top with grilled chicken.

Week 1, Day 7
Breakfast
1 cup oatmeal
¼ cup dried cranberries

Snack
4 graham crackers
1 cup rice milk

Lunch
Tuna Pita Sandwich
10 baked corn chips, unsalted

Snack
1 slice *Peach Toast*

Dinner
1 to 2 cups *Thai-Style Pesto with Rice Pasta*

Snack
2 cups popcorn
1 cup strawberries

Nutrition Content For Day
Calories: 1570
Fat: 40 g, 8 g saturated
Carbohydrates: 244 g
Protein: 72 g
Potassium: 1086 mg
Phosphorus: 402 mg
Sodium: 1432 mg

Recipes For The Day
Tuna Pita Sandwich
Ingredients:
One regular pita bread
2 oz. Albacore tuna, packed in oil
2 to 4 tbsp. of hummus
2 to 3 slices of cucumber
2 slices of onion

Directions:
You can either cut pita in half, or gently cut a small part of the top, creating a "pocket." Fill the pocket in this order with hummus, tuna, cucumber slices, onion. Mayonnaise may be added if desired.

Peach Toast
Ingredients:
1 slice white bread
1 tbsp. cream cheese
½ peach, sliced

Directions:
Toast bread. Spread with cream cheese. Top with sliced peaches.

Thai-Style Pesto with Rice Pasta
Ingredients:
1 pound ground turkey
1 lb. rice pasta, penne or wide noodles
1/3 cup fresh basil leaves
¼ cup dried basil leaves
1 large cloves garlic, pasted
½ lime, juiced
½ Chili pepper, seeded
¼ cup extra-virgin olive oil
Olive oil, for drizzling

Directions:
Brown turkey, set aside. Bring a large pot of water to a boil. Add the pasta and cook to al dente. Save water for later. Place the fresh and dried basil, garlic, lime juice, and chili into a food processor and "pulse" into a paste. Drizzle in the extra-virgin

olive oil. Pour the pesto into a large bowl and add a splash of the saved pasta water. Drain the pasta, add pasta and meat to the sauce and toss to combine. Drizzle with olive oil.

Week 2, Day 1
Breakfast
2 waffles
1 tsp. butter
1 cup raspberries

Lunch
1 *Cajun Stuffed Pepper*

Snack
1 medium pear
1 cup rice milk

Dinner
Bagel Sandwich
1 cup strawberries

Snack
3 cups popcorn
½ cup applesauce

Nutrition Content For Day
Calories: 1405
Fat: 54 g, 20 g saturated
Carbohydrates: 197 g
Protein: 43 g
Potassium: 1467 mg
Phosphorus: 805 mg,
Sodium: 1503 mg

Recipes For The Day
Pancakes
Directions:
Make pancakes with rice, tapioca or potato flour. Use rice milk in place of cow or goat milk. You also can add ½ to 1 cup kidney-friendly fruit, maple syrup, jam, butter, cinnamon to pancakes.

Cajun Stuffed Peppers
(Serves 6)
Ingredients:
1 cup chopped roasted red peppers
6 fresh bell peppers
½ lb ground beef
½ lb ground pork
¼ cup hot water
1 medium onion, chopped
3 cups, cooked white rice
½ tsp black pepper
½ tsp lemon pepper
1 tbsp dried thyme
1 tbsp minced garlic

Directions:
Pre-heat oven to 350 degrees.
Bring large pot of water to boil and drop in bell peppers, boiling for 5 min before draining.
Prepare peppers by removing stem and removing seeds.
In a large skillet, cook ground meat over medium heat until browned
Add hot water, roasted red peppers, onions, garlic and spices, cook for 5 min
Add rice and stir to combine and cook for 3 min.
Remove from heat and stuff bell peppers, then put stuffed peppers in a baking dish and bake uncovered for 30 min
Serve with garnish of roasted red peppers

Bagel Sandwich
Ingredients:
1 onion bagel
1 to 2 tbsp. mayo
1 tbsp. feta cheese
¼ cup alfalfa sprouts
1 small to medium roasted pepper
1 thin slice red onion
1 fried egg

Directions:
Cut bagel in half. Top in this order, spread mayo, feta cheese, onion, egg and sprinkle some seasonings if desired.

Week 2, Day 2
Breakfast
1 peach
1 English Muffin with 1 scrambled egg
1 cup rice milk

Snack
4 ounces of yogurt with fruit

Lunch
1 to 2 cups *Vegetable Beef Soup*
2 pieces of Italian bread (1" wide); you can add oil-based dipping sauce

Snack
1 rice cake with 1 tablespoons of jam

Dinner
5 to 6 inch of ¼ a loaf of *Garlic Bread*
6 *Garlic Roasted Asparagus Spears*
2 oz. grilled salmon

Snack
3 cup unsalted popcorn

Nutrition Content For Day
Calories: 1343
Fat: 59, 18 g saturated
Carbohydrates: 148 g
Protein: 62 g
Potassium: 1946 mg
Phosphorus: 815 mg

Recipes For The Day
Beef Vegetable Soup
Ingredients:
1 pound ground lean beef (90/10)
1 to 1 ½ cup of low sodium beef broth
3 to 4 ½ cup of water
1 cup carrots, sliced
¼ tsp. ground black pepper
1 cup celery, sliced
½ cup red pepper, chopped
½ cup radishes
1 clove garlic, minced
1 tsp. dried basil leaves
½ cup onion, diced

Directions:
Brown beef, set aside.
In large saucepan, over medium-high heat, bring broth, red pepper, garlic, carrots, celery, onion, basil, radishes and black pepper to a boil. Simmer 10 minutes. Add beef.

Roasted Garlic Asparagus Spears
Directions:
Ingredients:
6 asparagus spears
Garlic powder
Black pepper
½ tsp. olive oil

Directions:
Heat oven to 400 degrees. Place asparagus on baking sheet. Top with spices. Drizzle with oil. Roast for 10-15 minutes.

Week 2, Day 3
Breakfast
4 inch bagel with butter
Blueberry Smoothie

Lunch
1 to 1 ½ cups *Boiled White Turnips & Vegetables* over
1 to 2 cups rice, season to desired taste
2 oz. grilled chicken

Snack
Peach Toast

Dinner
Beef Burger

Snack
1 cup *Fruit Salad*
1 oz. melba toast with 1 tbsp. cream cheese

Nutrition Content For Day
Calories: 1,636
Fat: 54 g, 23 g saturated
Carbohydrates: 221 g
Protein: 64 g
Potassium: 1444 mg
Phosphorus: 658 mg
Sodium: 2036 mg

Recipes For The Day
Fruit Salad
Ingredients:
½ medium apple, diced in small pieces
½ cup blueberries
½ cup blackberries
8 grapes
¼ cup raspberries
2 to 3 tbsp. grape juice
You can add honey or vanilla extract, if desired

Directions:
In a large bowl, combine all ingredients. Gently toss to coat all fruits. Keep in refrigerator and serve chilled.

Boiled White Turnips & Vegetables
Ingredients:
4 or 5 white turnips
½ cup diced onion
½ cup celery, chopped
2 tbsp. canola oil
¾ cup water

Directions:
Cut raw turnips in pieces and boil in water until tender. Mix in celery and onion and canola oil in the water. Cook until done. Add butter, toss lightly and put over rice.

Burger
Ingredients:
1 lean beef burger patty
1 hamburger bun
1 to 2 lettuce leaves
1 slice onion
Seasoning and condiments can be added, such as mayo, etc. (no ketchup or mustard)

Directions:
Place patty on hamburger bun, top with lettuce, onion, and seasonings/condiments. Close with other hamburger bun.

Blueberry Smoothie
Ingredients:
¾ cup blueberries
4 oz. low fat yogurt
12 to 14 oz. of rice or almond milk
1 tsp. of vanilla extract

Directions:
Place all in blender and combine until smooth.
You can add honey, essential amino acid powder, acacia fiber, oils especially fish and flaxseed.

Week 2, Day 4
Breakfast
French Toast
You can add butter, maple syrup, etc.
Fruit Salad
1 cup rice milk

Snack
1 small roll toasted with 2 tablespoon jam

Lunch
Turkey Roll-ups
1 cup watermelon

Snack
1 c raspberries

Dinner
1 to 2 cups *Apple Bulgur Wheat Salad*
2 oz. grilled pork chop
½ cup steamed squash

Snack
Vanilla Wafer Dessert

Nutrition Content For The Day
Calories: 1563
Fat: 47 g, 16 g saturated
Carbohydrates: 218 g
Protein: 57 g
Potassium: 2253 mg
Phosphorus: 666 mg
Sodium: 1657 mg

Recipes For The Day
French Toast
Ingredients:
1 cup rice milk
2 eggs

1 tsp. vanilla extract
Pinch nutmeg
6 slices bread of choice

Directions:
Set aside bread slices. Mix all the other ingredients in a shallow bowl. Dip the bread slices into the milk mixture and place on a nonstick griddle, until light brown on both sides. You can bake bread on a greased cookie sheet in a 400°F oven until light gold on both sides, turning once.

Turkey Roll Up
Ingredients:
4 10-inch flour tortillas
8 slices deli turkey
1 tbsp low-fat mayonnaise
2 oz low fat cream cheese at room temperature
2 tbsp cranberry sauce
Lettuce

Directions:
Place tortillas in paper towel and microwave for 30-45 seconds until tortillas are soft and warm.
Meanwhile, combine softened cream cheese, mayonnaise and cranberry sauce until well-blended.
Place tortillas on flat surface, spreading ¼ of cream cheese mixture onto each tortilla. Cover with 2 slices of turkey and large lettuce leaf. Roll up tortillas like taco and refrigerate until set.

Apple Bulgur Wheat Salad
Ingredients:
½ cup bulgur wheat
1 cup diced unpeeled apples
2 tbsp. chopped celery
2 tbsp. dried cranberries
2 tbsp. low-sodium oil/vinegar dressing

Directions:
Cook, rinse, and drain pasta according to package directions. In a medium bowl, combine the cooked pasta with the rest of the ingredients and toss lightly.

Vanilla Wafer Desserts
Ingredients:
8 vanilla wafers
1 tsp. butter
½ tsp. strawberry jam

Directions:
Spread 4 wafers with butter and jam. Top with remaining wafers to make 4 cookie sandwiches. Bake for 10 minutes at 275°F degrees. Let cool. Note: each cookie sandwich may be dipped in melted white chocolate after baking and cooling if desired.

Week 2, Day 5
Breakfast
1 cheese omelet
1 cup rice milk
2 plums

Snack
2 slice *Peach Toast*

Lunch
1 to 2 cups *Israeli Couscous with Roasted Summer Vegetables & Grilled Chicken*

Snack
1 rice cake with jam
Dinner
½ cup green beans
1 to 2 cups rice
2 oz. grilled steak (not eaten often)

Snack
1 *Honey Lemon Glazed Pear*

Nutrition Content For Day
Calories: 1404
Fat: 46 g, 21 g saturated
Carbohydrates: 207 g
Protein: 51 g

Potassium: 1687 mg
Phosphorus: 707 mg
Sodium: 958 mg

Israeli Couscous with Roasted Summer Vegetables & Grilled Chicken
Ingredients:
¾ cup low sodium chicken broth
1 cup water
1 ¼ cup Israeli couscous or regular couscous
walnut oil for drizzling
1 ½ large cloves garlic
1 tsp. whole white cumin
1 dried red chili pepper (optional)
2 cup chopped summer vegetables such as yellow squash, mushrooms, zucchini, onions
¼ cup chicken broth
1 tbsp. balsamic vinegar
1 pound grilled chicken

Directions:
Heat the broth to boiling in a small saucepan. Stir in the grains and lower the heat to a simmer. Cover and cook for about 10-14 minutes. Remove the lid and set aside.

On sheet pan, place garlic and summer vegetables. Season with spices. Drizzle with oil. Roast for 20-25 minutes or until tender and slightly browned on edges. Place in heated skillet. Add the cooked couscous and the ¼ cup of broth. Cook for another five minutes, stirring, until the broth has cooked off and the chard is fully wilted. Add seasonings, vinegar, chicken, and serve.

Honey Lemon Glazed Pear
Ingredients:
¼ cup melted butter
1/3 cup honey
4 medium ripe to firm pears
½ lemon (for zesting and juicing)

Directions:
Heat oven to 450°F degrees. Grate and juice lemon. You should have 3 to 4 tablespoons juice. In a small bowl, whisk together butter, honey, and the lemon juice.

Peel the pears if you like, but it is not necessary. Cut the pears in half lengthwise. Using a melon baller or a ½ teaspoon measuring spoon, neatly scoop out the core.

Place the pears in an 8 by 10 inch glass baking dish, pan or ceramic pan. Pour glaze mixture over the pears, allowing it to flow into the pan. In the cavity of each pear half, sprinkle some grated lemon zest.

Bake pears for 10 minutes, and baste with glaze. Bake for another 10 minutes, or until pears are very tender. Baste again with glaze and cool slightly. Serve warm.

Week 2, Day 6
Breakfast
1 serving of *Overnight Oats*
1 cup rice milk

Snack
1 cup strawberries
8 vanilla wafers

Lunch
Grilled Steak (not to be eaten often) and Vegetable Wrap

Snack
5 to 10 pretzels
6 to 8 *Dried Apple Rings*

Dinner
2 oz. *Chicken with Herbs*
1 cup *Rice Pilaf*
1 cup steamed carrots

Snack
4 to 5 pieces of *Rice Crispy Clusters*

Nutrition Content For Day
Calories: 1690
Fat: 54 g, 13 g saturated
Carbohydrates: 252
Protein: 56 g
Potassium: 1607 mg
Phosphorus: 621 mg
Sodium: 1729

Recipes For The Day
Overnight Oats
Ingredients:
½ cup regular oats
1 cup rice milk, and more if needed
½ cup blueberries
½ cup blackberries
¼ tsp. pure vanilla extract

Directions:
Mix together all ingredients in a bowl and place in fridge overnight. In the morning, add your desired toppings and serve without heating.

Grilled Steak Wrap
Ingredients:
1 10-inch wrap
2 oz. grilled steak
1 to 2 tbsp. of matchstick cut carrots
1 to 2 tbsp. sliced seeded cucumber
1 to 2 tbsp. grated radishes
1 to 2 tbsp. low sodium ranch dressing

Directions:
Place wrap in a greased, heated skillet. Top with ranch dressing, vegetable, steak, and vegetables on halve of wrap. Close wrap with unused portion of wrap. Cook on both sides until golden brown.

Chicken w/ Herbs
(Serves 4-5)
Ingredients:
1 lb. chicken legs, thighs and breasts, skin removed
3 tbsp olive oil
3 tbsp balsamic vinegar
½ cup shallots, chopped
2 tsp dried thyme
2 tsp dried rosemary
½ tsp black pepper

Directions:
Rinse and pat chicken dry. Pour olive oil in a 12x8 inch baking dish, placing chicken in dish and lightly coating all surfaces with oil.
Sprinkle with vinegar, shallots and half the herbs.
Roast chicken in preheated 400 degree oven, uncovered for 20 min.
Turn chicken and sprinkle remaining herbs over it.
Increase oven temp to 425 degrees and roast additional 20 minutes. Serve.

Rice Pilaf
(Makes 4 Servings.)
Ingredients:
½ cup rice
1 cup sodium-free chicken broth
2 tsp olive oil
½ large onion, chopped
2 tbsp fresh parsley, chopped

Directions:
Bring rice and broth to a boil in medium saucepan. Reduce heat to low, covering and allowing rice to absorb liquid for about 15 min.
Heat oil in large skillet over medium heat, adding onion and stirring occasionally until onion browns, about 5 min.
Once rice is finished, fluff with fork and transfer to serving bowl. Stir in onion, parsley and season with pepper to taste.

Rice Crispy Clusters
Ingredients:
1 10-ounce bag of marshmallows
2 tbsp. butter
1 ½ cup rice crispy cereal

Directions:
Prepare a baking sheet by lining it with waxed paper; set aside. Microwave marshmallows and butter in a microwave safe bowl on high power for 2 to 3 minutes, stirring once or twice.

Stir in cereal and mix well. Drop by teaspoon onto prepared baking sheet and let cool until firm. Can be stored in an air tight container for up to 3 weeks.

Week 2, Day 7
Breakfast
1 *Italian-Style Cheese Omelet*

Snack
1 cup Blueberry Dream

Lunch
Tuna Pasta Salad
1 cup carrot sticks
1 tbsp. low-sodium dressing

Snack
1 apple
½ to ¾ cup cereal

Dinner
1 cup boiled kidney-friendly vegetables over
1 to 2 cups of pasta with garlic and oil
2 oz. roasted pork tenderloin

Snack
1 cup *Strawberry Lemonade Granita*

Nutrition Content For Day
Calories: 1235
Fat: 41 g, 10 g saturated
Carbohydrates: 167 g
Protein: 51 g
Potassium: 2350 mg
Phosphorus: 729 mg
Sodium: 815 mg

Recipes For The Day
Italian-Style Cheese Omelet
Ingredients:
2 slices turkey bacon
2 tbsp part skim ricotta cheese
2 tbsp fresh basil, chopped
3 eggs
1 tbsp water
2 tsp olive oil
2 tbsp parmesan cheese, grated

Directions:
Chop bacon, combining with basil and ricotta cheese in small mixing bowl. Stir to combine and set aside.
In separate mixing bowl, combine eggs, water and pepper, beating until combined.
In a 9-inch nonstick skillet add 2 tsp olive oil and swirl to cover. Add egg mixture and cook over medium heat until bottom of omelet is set and lightly browned, about 1-2 min.
Spoon bacon and cheese mixture onto half of omelet, using spatula loosen omelet around edges.
Fold omelet in half using spatula, sprinkle with parmesan and serve.

Blueberry Dream
Ingredients:
1 cup blueberries
1 cup vanilla yogurt
1 cup non-dairy frozen whipped topping

Directions:
Mix all together. Freeze.

Tuna Pasta Salad
(Serves 4)
Ingredients:
8 oz cooked rotini pasta
3 diced radishes
¼ cup chopped, peeled jicama
¼ cup diced water chestnuts
1 can white tuna fish
1 tbsp chopped fresh chives
Dressing:
2 tbsp lemon juice
1 ½ tsp low sodium dijon mustard
1 tsp canola oil
1/8 tsp minced garlic
1/8 tsp black pepper

Directions:
Drain tuna.
In large bowl, combine all dressing ingredients with whisk.
Add remaining ingredients to dressing, combining well.
Refrigerate for at least 1 hr. and serve chilled.

Strawberry Lemonade Granita
Ingredients:
2 ¼ cup water
½ cup sugar
½ cup fresh lemon juice (from 1 ½ lemons)
½ cup puréed strawberries

Directions:
In a medium saucepan, bring water and sugar to a simmer over medium-high heat until sugar is dissolved. Remove from heat; add lemon juice and strawberry purée.

Pour mixture into a shallow pan or dish and put in the freezer. Stir every 30 minutes with a fork until all of the liquid is frozen. Remove from freezer 20 to 30 minutes before serving.

Guides to Use with All 3 Diets

The following pages contain guides or information that can be used with any diet plan you have. It will be covering water and hydration, eating out guides for all 3 diets, cooking techniques to lower potassium, blanching olives and how to read a food label.

The Importance of Water & Hydration

Staying hydrated is important for everyone, but especially so when it comes to kidney disease. Being dehydrated can cause kidney damage leading to kidney disease.

Before following any of the hydration recommendations, check with your medical doctor to make sure you don't have any fluid restrictions. For some people with kidney disease there may be fluid restrictions that need to be adhered to.

As the kidney draws on water to be able to perform its filtration effectively, it's vital that you drink half your body weight in ounces of water daily. Herbal teas can count towards your water consumption.

It is best to spread out your water consumption throughout the day to provide your kidney the water it needs to properly function.

Calculation For Water Consumption

Body Weight divided by 2 = amount of ounces of water per day.

Eating Out With Kidney Disease

Having kidney disease doesn't necessarily mean you can't ever go out to eat. There are just certain extra precautions you must take to ensure that your good time out is as easy on your kidneys as possible.

Here are some general tips, everyone with CKD should keep in mind before eating out:

- Lay out a plan beforehand

- Look up the restaurant menu online to find options that are in line with kidney-friendly foods.

- If you are planning to incorporate sodium or potassium in your meal choices, try to refrain from dishes, which contain them earlier in the week.

- Try to make it a point to leave half of your meal and take it home with you. Many portions are too large.

- Ask your server for recommendations and that special preparations be made with your food, such as 'no added salt,' etc.

- Request that your sauces, dressings, gravies, etc. be omitted or added on the side.

The Low Protein Guide To Eating Out

Don't be embarrassed by the fact that you or a family member are on a diet and need to restrict certain foods. If you aren't familiar with the restaurant's menu, you can visit them online (many upload their menus) or you can always call ahead.

Do not hesitate to ask for modifications of foods on the menu, for example, pasta with garlic and oil in lieu of a tomato-based sauce. Most restaurants are accustomed to customers' diet constraints or food allergies, and will be happy to accommodate.

You can often make very satisfying meals by being creative with the menu. You can order multiple side dishes, appetizers, and salads. Explore the menu thoroughly and ask the staff about any recommendations.

Low Protein Choices at Restaurants

- **Japanese** – vegetable sushi, rice, rice noodles, vegetable dishes.

- **Chinese** – rice, beans, noodles, vegetable dishes.

- **Mexican** – burrito without cheese, sour cream, guacamole, rice, chips, salad bar, beans.

- **Steak Houses** – french fries (not to be eaten often), potato, salad bar, vegetable dishes.

- **Middle Eastern** – pita bread, beans, babaganoush, vegetable dishes.

- **American** – vegetable dishes, salad bar, salads, bread, fruit, veggie burger, beans (try to find out how much protein is in it).

The Vegetarian Guide To Eating Out

- **Japanese** – vegetable sushi, rice, rice noodles, vegetable dishes (like seaweed salad). Try to incorporate soy products like miso soup, tofu and tempeh instead of meat or poultry.

- **Chinese** – rice, beans, noodles, vegetable dishes. Again, try to focus on soy-based dishes, many Chinese restaurants now provide vegetarian soy-substitute meat dishes that are made with tofu. Experiment with different dishes and try to eat steamed options as opposed to anything breaded, fried or in heavy sauces.

- **Mexican** – burrito without cheese, sour cream, guacamole, rice, chips, salad bar, beans. Specifically, kidney-friendly beans like black beans, garbanzo beans/chickpeas and pinto beans.

- **Steak Houses** – french fries (not to be eaten often), potato, salad bar, vegetable dishes, salads.

- **Middle Eastern** – pita bread, beans, babaganoush, vegetable dishes, hummus.

- **American** – vegetable dishes, salad bar, salads, bread, fruit, veggie burger, beans (try to find out how much protein is in the veggie burger).

The Academy of Nutrition & Dietetics Guide To Eating Out

The Academy's kidney diet is a favorite for many people when it comes to eating out. It has many more options to choose from. Below we cover many options that are available to you.

American
- **Good breakfast choices** include eggs (no cheese), French toast, English muffin, hot cereal, bagel, or toast. Limit salty meats such as ham, sausage, and bacon.
- **Appetizer:** Choose plain wings or tossed salad instead of salted fried foods or potatoes.
- **Main Course:** Select unsalted lean beef, turkey, pork, chicken or seafood that is prepared baked, broiled, roasted, or grilled.
- **Side Dish:** Order kidney healthy vegetable options, such as, asparagus, green beans, corn, cooked cauliflower or carrots, coleslaw, macaroni salad, rice or a dinner roll. Forego potatoes or sweet potatoes, if limiting potassium.
- **Dessert:** Opt for sherbet, apple or blueberry pie, angel food cake, or a cookie without nuts or chocolate.

Fast Food
The majority of fast food options are high in sodium, potassium, and phosphorus, so you will need to prepare by making careful food choices the rest of the day or weekend.
- Choose a plain hamburger, grilled chicken sandwich, or sandwich (without cheese or sauce) or a salad.
- Ask for a vegetable, fruit, or side salad, instead of French fries.
- Order a small non-cola beverage, if any. Do not avail yourself of any free re-fill options.

Italian
- **Appetizer:** Choose salad or unsalted bread. Soups and antipasto can be high in sodium.
- **Main Course:**

- If you need to limit potassium, choose pasta with pesto, garlic and butter, or olive oil sauces **on the side**, instead of tomato-based sauces.
- Choose unsalted beef, veal, chicken and shellfish. Prosciutto, Italian sausage, and pepperoni are high in sodium
- If you order pizza, a slice without meat may be best along with a side salad.
- **Side Dish:** If you need to limit potassium, beware of tomatoes, cooked spinach, squash, potatoes or nuts.
- **Dessert:** Choose biscotti, Italian ice, almond cake, fruit tart, or a plain pastry instead of desserts made with custard, milk, or nuts.

Greek

- **Appetizer:** Limit olives, anchovies, fried calamari, and cheese or spinach-filled pastries.
- **Main Course:** Choose unsalted, grilled fish, chicken, lamb, or beef. Gyros, souvlaki, moussaka, or pastitsio may be high in sodium.
- **Side Dish:** Ask for a Greek salad but limit the tomatoes, feta cheese, olives, and capers.
- **Dessert:** Try diples (pastries with honey), sponge or lemon cake, or butter cookies, instead of those made with custard, milk, or nuts.

Asian

Many Asian foods and sauces are high in sodium. Request that all sauces be **on the side** and **no MSG** is used. Opt for ginger, hot pepper or chili oil to add flavor to your dish instead of soy sauce or fish sauces.

- **Appetizer:** Choose a tossed salad, pot stickers, chicken wings, or spring rolls. Skip the soups since they are often high in sodium.
- **Main Course:** Choose grilled meats and vegetables or tempura fried foods, but limit the high-sodium sauces.
- Order meats, fish or shell fish that are cooked. Sushi and sashimi includes raw fish or seafood which increases your risk of food-borne illness.
- **Side Dish:**
  - White rice is a better choice than fried rice.

- If you need to limit potassium, choose vegetables such as green beans, cabbage, carrots, onions, peppers, snow peas, and water chestnuts.
- **Dessert:** Fortune cookies.

Mexican
- **Appetizer:** Request unsalted tortilla chips. Salsa, guacamole, bean, and cheese dips are very high in sodium and potassium, so avoid them.
- **Main Course:** Select beef, chicken, seafood, or vegetarian tacos, burritos, enchiladas, tostadas, taquitos/flautas, or fajitas. Ask for beans and toppings **on the side**.
- **Side Dish:** Opt for white rice, lettuce, sautéed onions and bell peppers, and flour tortillas. Limit beans, refried beans, cheese, and Spanish/Mexican Rice.
- **Dessert:** Try apple enchiladas, sopapillas, or churros.

Cooking Techniques to Lower Potassium

Leaching & Double Cooking Method to Take Potassium Out of Foods

The process of leaching and double cooking will help pull potassium out of certain high potassium foods. This is referring to vegetables and potatoes. If you have high potassium levels these cooking methods will help reduce the potassium content in some vegetable and potatoes.

This is an extra cooking step that can help, but if you find it difficult in your lifestyle it can be held off till later stages of kidney disease. As kidney disease progresses your blood work may indicate consuming less potassium in your diet.

How to Leach Vegetables

For potatoes, sweet potatoes, carrots, beets, rutabagas, and all vegetables:

1. Peel and place the vegetables in cold water, so they won't darken.

2. Slice the vegetables about 1/8 inch thick.

3. Rinse in warm water for a few seconds.

4. Soak for a minimum of two hours in warm water. Use ten times the amount of water to the amount of vegetables. If soaking longer, try to change the water every few hours.

5. Rinse under warm water again for a few seconds.

6. If steaming cook vegetables with five times the amount of water to the amount of vegetables.

Leaching squash, mushrooms, cauliflower, and frozen vegetables:

1. Allow frozen vegetable to thaw to room temperature and drain.
2. Rinse fresh or frozen vegetables in warm water for a few seconds.
3. Soak for a minimum of two hours in warm water. Use ten times the amount of water to the amount of vegetables. If soaking longer, change the water every four hours.
4. Rinse under warm water again for a few seconds.
5. Cook the usual way, but with five times the amount of water to the amount of vegetables.

Double Cooking Potatoes to Lower Potassium

People with kidney disease can still eat potatoes by using the double cooking technique to reduce potassium. Although potassium is not totally removed, it is lowered enough to safely include a small portion and keep your diet kidney friendly. Double cooking technique for reducing potassium in potatoes:

1. Peel potatoes and cut into thin slices, dice small, or shred for hash browns.
2. Place potato pieces in a pot of water and bring to a boil.
3. Drain water then add fresh water.
4. Bring water to a boil and cook potatoes until tender.
5. Drain water and prepare potatoes as desired.

Blanching Olives to Reduce Sodium Content

Blanching, or boiling and immediately submerging in cold water can reduce the sodium content of olives, but only boil for one to two minutes since boiling longer than two minutes can result in mushy olives.

How to Read a Food Label
Tips For People with Chronic Kidney Disease

If you have CKD, you may need to limit some nutrients in your diet such as sodium, phosphorus, or potassium. You should limit saturated and transfats, too. Read food labels to help make healthy food choices for your kidneys.

- Check the Nutrition Facts label for sodium and protein.
- Check the ingredient list for added phosphorus and potassium.
- Look for claims on the label, like "low saturated fat" or "sodium free."

What Should I Look for on the Nutrition Facts Label?

Look for **sodium** and **protein** on the Nutrition Facts label. Some Nutrition Facts labels will list **phosphorus** and **potassium**, but they do not have to be posted on the label.

What to Look for on the Ingredient List?

The ingredient list is usually located underneath or near the food label. Ingredients will be listed in order of the amount in the food. The food has the most of the first ingredient on the list, and the least is the last ingredient on the list.

1. Look for phosphorus, or for words with PHOS on the ingredient list. Many packaged foods have phosphorus. Choose different foods when the ingredient list has PHOS on the label.

Ingredients: Rehydrated potatoes (Water, Potatoes, Sodium acid pyro**phos**phate), Beef (Beef, Water, Salt, Sodium **phos**phate).

This ingredient list shows that the food has added phosphorus.

2. Look for potassium on the ingredient list. For example, potassium chloride can be used in place of salt in some packaged foods, like canned soups and tomato products. Limit foods with potassium on the ingredient list.

Ingredients: Tomato juice, Vegetable juice blend, Potassium chloride, Sugar, Magnesium, Salt, Vitamin C (Ascorbic acid), Citric acid, Spice extract, Flavoring, Disodium Inosinate, Disodium Guanylate.

This ingredient list shows that the food has added potassium. Look for Claims on Food Packages to Help You Find Kidney Friendly Foods:

- Saturated Fat Free
- Sodium Free
- Low Saturated Fat
- Very Low Sodium
- Less Saturated Fat
- Low Sodium
- Trans Fat Free
- Reduced Salt

Sodium chloride (salt) is replaced in some foods with potassium chloride. If you need to watch your potassium, check the ingredient list.

	Nutrition Facts	
The amount listed is for one 1 cup serving. If you eat two servings, the amounts double.	Serving Size: 1 cup (228g)	
	Servings Per Container: 2	This package has two 1 cup servings.
	Amount Per Serving	
	Calories: 260 **Calories from Fat:** 120	
	% Daily Value*	One serving has 28% Daily Value of sodium.
	Total Fat 13g — 20%	
	Saturated Fat 5g — 25 %	▪ 5% or less is low.
	Trans Fat 2g	
	Cholesterol 30mg — 10 %	▪ 20% or more is high.
One serving has 660 milligrams of sodium.	**Sodium** 660mg — 28 %	
	Total Carbohydrate 31g — 10%	For this food label, 28% Daily Value is high for sodium.
	Dietary Fiber 0g — 0 %	
	Sugars 5g	
One serving has 4 grams of protein.	**Protein** 4g	
	Vitamin A 4% Vitamin C 2%	
	Calcium 15% Iron	

* Percent Daily Values are based on a 2,000 Calorie Diet

Baking & Bread Making

Baking your own bread, muffins and grain products to limit or eliminate sodium and protein has been a way to help kidney disease for decades. This can benefit anyone with kidney disease but can be reserved for later stages if blood work doesn't require stricter control over protein and sodium. However, there is no reason you can't begin doing this at any stage, as earlier interventions usually show a better outcome.

Any commercial bread making machines on the market will have instructions for how to bake breads. There are many books and online recipes for baking with lower protein flours. Do your best to limit or replace the sugar with honey or maple syrup and minimize or eliminate egg use.

Final Thoughts

Thank you again for purchasing this program!

I hope this book was able to help you to improve your kidney disease as it did mine.

The next step is to begin whichever diet you think is best for you given your situation, stick to it and see the results on your next blood work. You also have the option of combining diets for your lifestyle and preferences.

Remember, even if you aren't a 100% on the diet you've chosen, you can still benefit from it and if you happen to have a bad meal or snack, just begin the diet again the next time you eat.

Also, be sure to visit our website at http://www.healthykidneyinc.com which has hundreds of free articles, videos, our products and services to further support kidney health. Use discount code: healthykidney30 for 30% off any purchase.

You can also find our products on amazon.com. Search, "Kidney Restore and Kidney Shield" to learn more.

If you have any questions, need assistance in helping with food options or anything at all please contact us and we are happy to assist you.